THE FOOD COMBINING DIET

About the Author

Kathryn Marsden trained originally in hotel management which sparked her all-consuming interest in nutrition and food science. When her husband Ralph was diagnosed with cancer, she embarked upon an ambitious study of different dietary treatments to try to help him and became so enthralled by the fascinating potential of simple food substances in treating disease that she turned her attention full-time to the health, beauty and fitness field.

Kathryn went on to qualify as a nutritionist and continues to run a busy practice dealing with requests for help from people with a diverse number of illnesses and stress-related conditions. Her studies included physiology, anatomy, biology, biochemistry and the naturopathic and orthomolecular approaches to nutrition. She holds a Diploma in Clinical Nutrition and Nutritional Counselling. Also a freelance journalist, Kathryn has her own regular columns in professional, health and popular magazines and contributes regularly to a range of other publications.

She is a familiar voice on BBC, local and independent radio and television. She is a member of the Faculty of the The Tisserand Institute and teaches nutrition to students at the Royal Masonic Hospital and at Colleges of Further Education. Much in demand as an after dinner speaker, she gives lectures and seminars nationwide.

When she is not travelling, Kathryn returns to her home base in rural Wiltshire. She is a keen gardener and is ably assisted by her rescued cats, Sophie and Sylvester.

THE FOOD COMBINING DIET

Lose Weight the Hay Way

KATHRYN MARSDEN

Thorsons

An Imprint of HarperCollinsPublishers

To my husband Ralph

For enriching so many lives
with your courage, loyalty,
love and laughter

Thorsons
An Imprint of HarperCollins*Publishers*
77–85 Fulham Palace Road
Hammersmith, London W6 8JB
1160 Battery Street,
San Francisco, California 94111–1213

Published by Thorsons 1993
13 15 17 19 20 18 16 14

A catalogue record for this book
is available from the British Library

ISBN 0 7225 2790 X

Phototypeset by Harper Phototypesetters Limited,
Northampton, England
Printed and bound in Great Britain by
Caledonian International Book Manufacturing Ltd, Glasgow

Contents

Contents

Acknowledgements

Without these people, the writing and researching of this book would have been much more difficult, perhaps impossible, to undertake.

My grateful thanks go to:

Dr John Stirling for his patience and valuable advice throughout the preparation and writing stages of the *Food Combining Diet* and for spending so much time in minutely checking my manuscript. His command of the science of Food Combining is inestimable. I will also be eternally grateful for the support, friendship and professional help he gave so willingly — and which made so much difference — during Ralph's recovery.

Carolyn Hill, Senior Nutritionist at Waitrose, Bracknell and her colleagues for providing so much information on food values, product labelling and ingredients — and for never once making me feel that I was taking up too much of their time.

Malmesbury Library. The Head Librarian and staff are truly wonderful. No matter how obscure or difficult my research requests, they always managed to find the answers to my questions. An example in courtesy and kindness.

Caroline Wheater, who put me on the book writing trail in the first place.

Sarah Sutton at Thorsons for her cheerfulness and encouragement.

Shirley Mathias at Wiltshire Newspapers — she's a star.

Isabel Moore for her cookery expertise.

Jan and Tony Robinson for opening their home and their hearts to me, providing an oasis of comfort and cheer on my many exhausting journeys.

Gillian Hamer, for her friendship, encouragement and inspiration.

Of course to Jean Joice, whose best-selling *Food Combining For Health*, written with Doris Grant, has made so much difference to so many people. Special thanks for all her letters, notes, tips and welcome advice.

Muriel Dubourdieu, whose talent at second-hand book finds allowed me to read so much without going bankrupt. Her benevolence and lovely smiling face have brightened many a day. She alone was responsible for the publication of my very first magazine article.

Ralph, my long-suffering husband, for the time he has taken in checking, rechecking and editing my manuscript and for helping with the project in so many other ways.

Thank you all.

Foreword

Originally I had certain misgivings about the use of the word 'diet' in the proposed title of Kathryn Marsden's book about Food Combining — since it implies something you go on and in due course come off, whereas the Hay System is essentially a way of life. However, all doubts were dispelled when I read her completed manuscript. She graphically describes how weight loss achieved the Hay way also improves health and spirits to a remarkable degree, and her ideas are solidly backed by meticulous research and expertise based on practical experience with the many patients she has helped over the years.

For it is a curious paradox that people who embark on the Hay System because they have health problems invariably find that, if overweight, they also lose their surplus pounds without even trying.

Conversely, overweight people who have failed with so-called slimming diets and turn to the Hay system find that not only do they lose weight, but instead of feeling miserable and deprived feel better and more energetic than they have for years.

People who enjoy buoyant health do not usually have weight problems, since given ideal conditions the body will regulate itself and shed any surplus that prevents it functioning at peak level.

As Dr Hay put it almost sixty years ago, 'Just as soon as we cease causing disease, nature starts in at once to readjust things to normal and she will always succeed if we continue to allow her to work unhampered.'

By this he meant separating foods that do not digest well together so that the body can use the food we eat more efficiently and without 'clogging the system'.

That this simple formula for health really works has been endorsed in the many enthusiastic letters that Doris Grant and I have received since the publication of our book *Food Combining for Health*. Although written primarily to introduce a new generation of readers to the benefits of compatible eating — freedom from headaches, indigestion, arthritis, irritable bowel syndrome and in Sir John Mills' case duodenal ulcer — the recurrent theme of the letters has been how well their writers feel for the first time in years and how surplus pounds have melted away in the course of their recovery from whatever was troubling them.

During the course of preparation Kathryn and I have had several lively discussions about many of the issues she raises and I have been enormously impressed by the thoroughness and integrity of her work. *The Food Combining Diet* will not only be a boon to weightwatchers, but a welcome and rewarding addition to the bookshelves of all Hay enthusiasts. I wish it and its author every possible success.

Jean Joice

Preface

━━━━━━━━━━━━ ❧ ━━━━━━━━━━━━

' "You must sit down", says Love, "and taste my meat."
So I did sit and eat.'

George Herbert (1593–1633)
English poet of the Metaphysical School

I first became acquainted with my husband Ralph in 1975 via
a B.B.C. radio broadcast and, as a result of this introduction,
we corresponded for a while before actually meeting. The
consequence of love at first letter became love at first sight and
romance blossomed. The critics were flummoxed. Late
marriage to a middle-aged man nearly 20 years my senior raised
an eyebrow or two but we were never in any doubt about its
constancy. He had suffered for years from stress, living out of
a suitcase, travelling, paying little attention to diet and putting
on too much weight, resulting eventually in diabetes. In fact,
one of my first major excursions into nutritional therapy was
the reading of eleven books on diabetes in as many days. I was
totally fascinated. We joined the British Diabetic Association,
corresponded regularly with their incredibly helpful medical
advisers and bought and read still more books. Food, I began
to recognize, was indeed a science as well as sustenance for the
soul. This was valuable experience, but still not enough to
prepare me for what was to come.

When Ralph was diagnosed subsequently with cancer it seemed, at the time, to be the cruellest blow life could assign. He underwent two major operations, one for the complete removal of his stomach and a second which divorced him from his spleen. Kept alive by a drip for about five weeks, he was discharged into my care with the (private) words (to me) that I should not be too hopeful of any recovery.

It was only when it came to dressing him for the journey home that I realized how frail he had become. His weight had dropped from 225 lb to 126 lb (that's 16 stones to 9 stones) — and to keep his trousers from falling down I had to tie them with hospital tape around his almost non-existent waist. Doing his best to cheer *me* up, Ralph joked that the hospital was keeping his insides but throwing the patient away.

Learning how to feed someone who has no stomach and no interest in food certainly concentrates the mind. Everything we tried made him sick — even water until we discovered he was ultra-sensitive to chlorine and began to filter it.

Sympathy and kindness were shown to us in abundance but there was a dearth of practical help. Even the technologically astounding surgery was no match for a shattered immune system and a frail body. What happens to food if the stomach has been taken away? And how could Ralph be properly nourished by what was turning out to be a very limited diet? Consultations and correspondence with medical experts, dietitians, medical charities and self-help groups produced nothing more than 'Don't worry' and 'I'm sure he'll be fine' but anyone could see that they didn't really believe it.

I still have the guidelines written by a hospital dietitian as to Ralph's suggested meal requirements. 'He is to eat plenty of sausages and bacon, margarine on bread and potatoes, cakes, scones, to drink lemonade and not to worry about fruits and vegetables because they are low in calories'! Any suggestions I made about digestive difficulty or malabsorption syndrome were cast aside as 'unlikely'. I don't believe that the doctors were being deliberately obstructive or awkward; they were simply reluctant to consider anything remotely connected with nutrition.

The first glimmer of light came from across the Pond. The Americans were – and, I believe, still are – light years ahead of the UK with their studies into nutritional therapy. The fellow-feeling and generosity were overwhelming. Correspondence came and went from nutritionists, writers, doctors and universities. I pored over the work of Adelle Davies, whose recommendations on vitamins and minerals, hydrochloric acid (people without stomachs don't have any), Vitamin B12 (likewise), digestive enzymes and acidophilus were breakthroughs of lifesaving proportions.

It was during this burning of much midnight oil that I came across a 1935 edition of a book called *Health Via Food* by Dr William Howard Hay; my first introduction to food combining. This was a 'find' which brought further amazing improvements. Little by little, as every spare inch of wall space gave way to bookshelves, Ralph gained in strength. The ashen face and sallow skin were replaced by a healthy glow, the discomfort lessened and he observed 'people stopped expecting me to snuff it'. Apart from limited mobility caused by the extensive surgery and resultant scar tissue, Ralph continues to be well. Looking after someone who clearly suffered a great deal of pain and discomfort but never once complained has, for me, been a humbling experience; an honour and an education. I revel in a continuing learning process that shows me, time and time again, the common sense and wisdom of Mother Nature, the amazing power of natural medicine and of shrewd, enjoyable eating.

In my work as a nutritionist I have seen many, many patients with a wide variety of problems, some acute, some chronic, some more serious than others but all significant. Overweight, underweight, arthritic, diabetic, insomniac, anxious, depressed, hypertensive, hypoglycaemic and constipated. Crohn's disease, heart disease, Raynaud's disease, colitis, indigestion, migraine, pre-menstrual syndrome — the very great majority have responded to simple, sensible changes to diet. By not mixing foods that fight, those with weight problems have lost stubborn and excess pounds with more ease than they thought possible. I am grateful to so many of them for the help and encouragement they gave me and for believing that the help I offered them was worthwhile enough to warrant inclusion in any book. Without their urging, their inspiration and their cheer, this book would probably never have been written. I'm convinced that you will find the Food Combining Diet as valuable as they have and hope that you will enjoy it as much as I have enjoyed researching and writing it!

Kathryn Marsden
Malmesbury, Wiltshire, England
June 1992

How to Use This Book

~

The Food Combining Diet brings Dr Hay's teachings right up to date and incorporates them into a no-hassle 28-day menu plan. It is the ultimate weight control programme for busy people who have no time for counting calories, calculating allocations or concocting complex cuisine. Even if extra pounds are not your problem, the book can also be used as an introduction to food combining – a first step to finding out more about the Hay way and its amazing health-giving gifts.

In preparing the Food Combining Diet, I have deliberately avoided elaborate, time-consuming recipes and opted for simple fare. Not only are the menus easy to follow, they are quick to prepare, flexible and interchangeable too. And many of the salads, soups and light meals make great travelling food or lunchtime meals for the office.

The Food Combining Diet also has a built-in cleansing programme which helps to improve elimination of toxins. You will see that the meals on Friday evening, Saturday breakfast and Saturday lunch are predominantly alkaline-forming fresh fruits and vegetables, extra low in protein and fat. But you won't feel hungry because intake is never restricted. You can eat as much as you like. If you do feel peckish between meals, enjoy an extra piece of fruit, some crunchy crudités, a handful of sunflower or pumpkin seeds or a glass of fresh juice. If there is a particular food amongst the menus which is not to your taste, then feel free to exchange it for something else as long as it is within the same category (i.e. change protein for protein or starch for starch). The Quick Reference Chart will guide you.

The availability of fresh fruits, vegetables and salads will depend upon the season and the part of the world in which you live but there is no need to restrict yourself to just two or three items. Choose as wide a variety as possible from the lists provided.

When you discover the lasting benefits of food combining and want to discover more, take a look at the recommended reading section at the back of this book.

Above all, remember that the Food Combining Diet is all about enjoying your meals and balancing your weight sensibly, safely and forever.

Why Dieting Doesn't Work

'A wonderful bird is the pelican;
His bill will hold more than his belican.
He can take in his beak
Food enough for a week
But I'm darned if I see how the
helican.'

The Pelican *by Dixon Lanier Merritt*
(1879–1954)

If you are thinking about following the Food Combining Diet, chances are you've dieted before. The 'Miracle Diet'; The 'Ultra Slim Diet'; The 'Lose 10 lb in 10 Days Diet'; The 'Give Up And Suffer Diet'; The 'I Can't Stand It Any Longer, I Must Have A Piece Of Chocolate Diet'. You've probably tried them all. Either you lost weight but have put it back on again or you found low calorie dieting too difficult to follow and gave up. One way or another, the diet failed. But you didn't fail — so don't feel badly about it. It's not your fault that each new regime turned out to be even more dreadful than the one before. By their very nature, short-term, start-stop-start weight loss diets are doomed to disaster before they begin.

So you lost 7 pounds? Big deal. You were permanently hungry, you felt terrible and, as soon as you packed it in, you put on 8 pounds! Shedding half a stone in a week may seem spectacular until you realize that what you lost, so impressively and dramatically during the first few days, was mostly only water and a substance called glycogen (a reserve energy source made from glucose and released by the liver to maintain blood sugar levels). If you shed any fat at all, it was probably only a couple of pounds.

So Why Do We Do It?

Started by the 1920s flappers and reinforced by the flat-chested cat walkers of the 60s, striving to be thin is a modern Western idea, preserved by the dictates of fashion houses and advertisers who would have us believe that carrying even a surplus ounce means we will miss out. But miss out on what? Nothing good, that's for sure. Repeated low calorie dieting is a risky business; it's also boring and unhealthy.

What Does 'Diet' Really Mean?

Dictionary references define the word 'diet' in two ways: firstly, as 'a way of feeding'; the food a person needs each day to remain healthy and sustained. The second definition, the one we use most commonly in everyday conversation, is 'to slim'; also to 'feed on special food as a regimen or punishment'. The term 'punishment' is well suited to the modern use of the word 'diet' — an inflexible, cheerless, deplorable and miserable way of eating less for the sole purpose of trying to lose weight.

Dieting is deprivation. It loads you up with stress and anxiety and robs you of nourishment and pleasure.

The Food Combining Diet couldn't be more different!

This book shows you how you can lose weight happily and healthily without counting or cutting calories ever again! It's a way of eating for a healthy life. Most important of all, it works.

Deprivation Dieting Can Damage Your Health

Habitual dieting usually involves a see-saw of compulsive calorie counting punctuated by throwing caution to the winds. This pattern can hurl your hormones out of kilter, derange your metabolic rate, aggravate existing health problems, devastate your resistance to disease and increase the likelihood of serious illness.

The more deprivation diets you follow, the heavier you become.

Years on the dieting yo-yo can also make you fat. Starving the body means starving the brain and disturbing the delicate feedback mechanism which controls appetite. Any dramatic reduction in food intake is recognized as a threat and so the system takes action to slow down your metabolic rate in order to save energy. When you begin to eat normally again, your energy burner is still idling. Your increased food supply simply doesn't get burned off. The pay-back for all your trouble and determination is that you have gained more pounds than you lost but, in the process, forfeited your vitality, energy and well-being.

Research suggests that although the dieter's metabolic rate undoubtedly falls on a low calorie regime, it can recover given the right circumstances. The Food Combining Diet provides you with a thoroughly enjoyable way of eating which maintains that all-important metabolic balance.

Calorie Counting Is Dead

Or it should be. Calorie counting has become such an obsession that some dieters won't eat anything until they have consulted their state-of-the-art credit-card-sized calorie calculators. Unfortunately, this misguided habit simply perpetuates the most significant problem suffered by all professional dieters — undernourishment.

The Food Combining Diet is successful without cutting calories; or counting them. It doesn't need to.

Most weight loss diets remind the long-suffering dieter, with monotonous frequency, that in order to weigh less you must eat less. To be slimmer, you have to reduce calories. You are warned that any food which isn't burned off as energy will end up as fat. *You* end up feeling really guilty about those extra few pounds. After all, aren't you overweight because you ate too much? In my experience as a practitioner, this is rarely the case and it is insulting to those who make every effort to eat healthily but still stay stubbornly chubby. Sure, there are bound to be some people who overeat and, as a consequence, carry excess weight. But there are also lots of people who have enormous appetites and never put on an ounce. And I've met plenty of plump people who exist hungrily on a sparrow's diet and don't lose any weight at all.

There Is More to a Weight Problem Than Just Overeating

I believe that it's time we looked more closely at the reasons for obesity and questioned the simplistic idea that weight gain follows on automatically from overeating. My own observations would seem to suggest that plump people metabolize their food at different rates from lean people, even when both groups are eating similar amounts of calories.

In addition, there are the problems of overweight in relation to undetected disease in general and hormonal imbalances in particular. For example, an underactive thyroid gland can be the cause of obstinate obesity. Unfortunately, the orthodox parameters for testing thyroid function are wide and fallible so that this common illness can go undiagnosed and untreated. In my experience, many sad sufferers of hypothyroidism (an underactive thyroid gland) are still being advised by their doctors to 'eat less and you'll weigh less'. Unfortunately, for these people, all the low-calorie diets in the world won't shift their extra pounds if they continue to remain undernourished.

Whilst heredity may play some part in determining the efficiency of the thyroid gland, another cause of malfunction is inadequate nutrition and poor absorption due to faulty digestion and, if my observations of patients are anything to go by, a sluggish liver. Aim for good health and weight control will follow.

We tend to equate being malnourished with eating too little but an overweight body can be just as under-supplied with nutrients as one which is too thin.

A moderately active adult needs a daily supply of around 1800-2000 kilocalories if he or she is to stay healthy and be properly nourished. Reduce the calories below this level for any length of time and you reduce the number of healing nutrients needed by the body for repair and rejuvenation.

The Food Combining Diet Nurtures and Heals

The wonderful advantage of Food Combining is that it does seem to have the ability to rectify so many disease states. Although the scientific reasons for its tremendous healing powers have yet to be explored, my feeling is that Food Combining, by improving digestion, absorption, metabolism and elimination, feeds the body with the nutrients it needs and thereby rebalances the whole system.

There is no boring, time-consuming calorie counting or microscopic weighing of every tiny morsel on the Food Combining Diet. You'll eat tasty, sustaining meals in satisfying amounts which will give you masses of energy *and* help you to reach your natural body weight.

How Much Weight Should I Expect to Lose?

You know already that any dramatic drop in weight triggered by low-cal dieting is a short-term con trick and that kilos lost quickly always creep back.

A patient of mine who came to me originally with chronic premenstrual syndrome and asked if I could help her weight problem lost two stones [28 lb/13 kilos] on the Food Combining Diet in just over three months. That's about 2 lb a week. The PMS has also vanished and the woman concerned is delighted with her new figure. When I met her again recently, she was reminiscing about one of the low-calorie diet plans she had followed before changing to the Food Combining Diet. 'I lost two stones in three weeks', she told me, 'and then put it all back on again in the following two weeks. What a waste of time! I'm so much happier with the Hay Way and I feel so different'.

By following the Food Combining Diet, you, too, can achieve a steady and maintained weight loss which, once gone, will stay gone. This is the safe, sensible way to slim so don't expect any sudden shedding of stones or kilos in the first few days. And if you are following the Food Combining ideal just for good health reasons but don't want to lose weight, you won't. That's the wonderful thing about it. Food Combining adjusts and then sustains your natural body weight.

What Happens If I Am Already Underweight?

Food Combining can help those who are underweight too. By improving digestion and absorption of food, the body becomes better nourished and weight better balanced.

> 'Some ladies smoke too much and
> Some ladies drink too much and
> Some ladies pray too much
> But all ladies think that they weigh too much.'
> Ogden Nash (1902-1971)
> American writer of humorous verse

Weight Moves In Mysterious Ways

Forget the bathroom scales. Apart from their being notoriously inaccurate and terribly touchy about creeping carpet pile and imperfect floorboards, bathroom scales can either delight or deflate you by registering as much as a 3 or 4 pound difference in weight between morning and evening. This is natural, applies to everyone and won't necessarily mean you lost or gained anything. It is also contrarily true that you can be very much aware of a significantly tighter or slacker waistband or belt without an inkling of confirmation from the wavering needle of your weighing machine.

So, if you weigh yourself at all, do it just once a week, at the same time of day, in the same state of dress or undress, with the scales in the same floor position. And then ignore the results!

Food Combining Simplified

The healthy eating innovation which has become known universally as 'Food Combining' is accredited to an inspired medical man called Dr William Howard Hay. At the age of only 40, already seriously overweight and in failing health, Dr Hay had been told by his physicians that his chances of recovery were limited. At that relatively tender age, he was suffering from Bright's disease (a serious kidney condition), high blood pressure and an enlarged heart; the medical services of the early 1900s could offer him nothing.

As is so often the case in perilous situations, necessity became the mother of invention. Dr Hay, spurred by the work of the early nature–cure practitioners, created a fundamentally uncomplicated way of eating which was to prove powerful enough to reduce his weight by 50 lb, to normalize his blood pressure and to eradicate his kidney and heart problems. The subsequent use of similar dietary guidelines with his own patients provided proof aplenty that Dr Hay's principles were correct. He was a modest man and never claimed to cure any illness or even to have discovered anything new; only that the simple dietary innovation which now bears his name merely allows Nature's own suppressed healing powers to surface.

Dr Hay believed that disease resulted from the accumulation of toxicity and acid waste products in the body and that this chemical imbalance was caused by four main factors:

1. Eating too many acid-forming proteins, starches and refined foods
2. Poor elimination of wastes and toxins
3. Eating too few of the beneficially alkaline-forming vegetables and fruits
4. Incompatible mixing of certain foods, in particular starches with proteins.

All these evils, Dr Hay proved, could be remedied by only a few elementary changes to daily routine:

1. Cut down on proteins, starches and highly processed foods
2. Improve elimination of acid wastes and toxins
3. Increase intake of vegetables, salads and fruits
4. Don't mix foods that fight.

I have had occasion to meet some people who have already tried Food Combining but who, sadly, gave up because they found it "complicated". Whilst there are a few important principles which need to be followed if the Hay Way is to succeed, no-one should abandon Food Combining as too difficult. It doesn't need to be *difficult*, it's just *different*. Food combining is the natural way. Consuming several different items from different food groups at one meal is a relatively modern habit and not always a healthy one. To appreciate why more careful food combinations are so important for good health, I think it really helps to understand a little of how the body deals with the tremendous variety of foodstuffs we load — often thoughtlessly — into it. Don't worry, I'm not going to bother you with endless anatomy and physiology; just follow me . . .

Most (misguided) mixed meals are made up of a starch (perhaps potato, rice, pasta, bread or other grains), a protein (maybe chicken, fish, eggs, cheese or milk), possibly a vegetable or two and then fruit — often as a dessert. All this is then mashed up and swallowed. Given that proteins take longer to digest than starches and that starches take longer than vegetables or fruits, mixing them together on the same plate or in the same mouthful can cause some people's digestive systems a great deal of grief. Have sympathy for those poor old enzymes and acids down there in the dark, trying to sort out the muddle of which stays in the stomach for several hours and which moves on more quickly to the next department.

In addition, it is a common misconception that digestion of all foods takes place in the stomach. In fact, starch (carbohydrate) breakdown begins in the mouth, initiated by a starch-splitting enzyme called ptyalin found in the alkaline juices of the saliva. The more thorough the chewing which takes place here, the better the digestion of the starchy food — a process which, if given the right circumstances — continues once those carbohydrates reach the stomach chamber.

Proteins move more slowly through the system and require an entirely different treatment. Whilst chewing is still important (for breaking protein down into swallowable proportions), nothing much else happens to it until the stomach acids are stimulated into action. Note the word "acids". Our starch, you will remember, needs an alkaline medium during the first stages of its journey.

Mix starches with proteins at the same meal and the digestive system won't know if it is functioning on acid foot or alkaline horseback.

The amount of processed and refined food which we eat can

also have a detrimental effect upon the efficiency of the digestion. Our hunter-gatherer ancestors certainly didn't indulge in the kind of mixed food fiasco we are familiar with today. Nor did they have coffee, cola, sugar, frozen T.V. dinners or take-aways. Obesity and cardiovascular disease were extremely rare. These peoples thrived on a nutrient-rich and high alkaline-forming diet which consisted predominantly of roots, shoots, nuts, berries and seeds (the gathered food) with some meat (the hunted food).[3]

Investigations have shown that the hunt was successful only 25 to 35 per cent of the time and this meant that the hunter-gatherer diet was made up of one third acid-forming meat and two-thirds alkaline-forming vegetable-based foods.[1] Meat may have been cooked on some kind of open fire, but was certainly not dragged back to camp or cave to be served with chips, gravy and soggy cabbage![2]

Anthropological and archaeological studies show that hunter gatherers had surprisingly successful health records supported by a nutritious diet not all that different from the official recommendations we are being encouraged to follow today.[3] But despite the ample evidence and plentiful publicity that we would all benefit from a healthier way of eating, it seems the majority of us still consume excessive amounts of protein and fat, not enough fibre and far too little fresh produce.[4,5]

Now I'm not suggesting that to succeed on the Food Combining Diet you must survive on raw meat or swap your supermarket trolley for hedgerow berries, but the criteria for reducing the amount of overcooked processed food and for increasing on natural and fibrous vegetables and fruits are sound.[6]

Raw salads, fruits and vegetables are packed with nourishment. Heating destroys important health-giving vitamins as well as enzymes which help digestion. The cooking water — usually thrown away — is also rich in nutrients such as potassium and magnesium.[7,8] As a result it is the plughole in the kitchen that is likely to be 'the best fed mouth in the house'. Raw salad and vegetable foods are frequently dismissed as difficult to digest but it is more often the incorrect combining of certain foods which causes discomfort rather than whether they are cooked or raw. However, the belief that to be healthy you must exist on a completely raw diet is absurd. Hot cooked meals bestow benefits upon the body which uncooked foods cannot. In the middle of winter, for example, we are sustained far more satisfyingly by thick nourishing soups and casseroles than by chilled salads! Moderation, variety and balance are the keys to eating healthily and well.

One of my main aims in writing this book is to bring enjoyable, healthy eating and effective weight loss to people who want to improve their diets but lead busy lives and have little time for the complexities normally associated with dieting. The Food Combining Diet explains the Hay formula in easy-to-follow language. All you need to do is begin by observing these simple rules and the rest will soon fall into place:

---

1. Don't mix starch foods or sugars with proteins.
2. Increase your intake of fresh vegetables, salads and fruit.
3. Keep all fruits away from main meals.
4. Don't mix milk with protein or starch.
5. Avoid processed, refined foods.

I always advise my own patients that, when altering their diets, changes should be made gently and slowly. Don't worry about becoming an expert at food combining overnight. Dr Hay counselled that any improvements should be introduced 'by degrees'. It is perfectly acceptable to begin by observing cardinal rules one and two: **Don't mix starches or sugary foods with proteins and Increase your intake of fresh produce.** Other modifications will fall into place in time, but if these first two recommendations are the only ones you are able to follow, you will still benefit.

Please do keep in mind the most important factor of all. The consuming of food may be vital for nourishing and fuelling the body but it is also supposed to be an enjoyable social activity. If a new way of eating doesn't seem to suit you or your lifestyle, don't stress your system by trying to follow it. As an American friend of mine is fond of saying: 'If a diet's a drag, don't do it!'

In any eating plan, watch out for the three Es:
EXCESSES, EXTREMES AND EXCLUSIONS.

If you read about something which is supposed to be good for you, don't go mad and eat it at every meal. On the other hand, the occasional enjoyment of a treat which is known to be less than nutritionally sound — a bar of chocolate, a sweet pastry or pizza, for example, can do wonders for a sagging psyche! It's the excesses which are potentially dangerous. So, enjoy your food, avoid going to extremes and remember — there is no need to exclude everything that's wicked!

The Food Combining Diet is:

For good health and well-being
For weight control and balance
Full of energy and vitality
Satisfying and enjoyable
Allows you to indulge!

The Dieter's Nightmare! Hypoglycaemia

If your attempts at losing weight have been accompanied by such unpleasant symptoms as dizziness, palpitations, anxiety, panic attacks, confused thinking, poor coordination, complete or sudden loss of energy, hollow stomach, extreme coldness, excessive perspiration during the day, hot or cold night sweats, a need for frequent meals, excessive thirst, drowsiness or unexplained emotional outbursts, you could be suffering from low blood sugar (hypoglycaemia). Often referred to as a 20th century epidemic, hypoglycaemia (hypo=low; glycaemia=blood glucose) is a condition where the levels of glucose in the blood fluctuate erratically and fall way below normal levels. And it's a problem extremely familiar to dieters. Hypo swings and sugar cravings are the two major reasons why diets are broken. You become so hungry and so desperate for food that you have to eat something, anything — and quickly!

How Does It Happen?

A body needing food first receives a message from a control centre in the brain. The level of glucose in your blood has fallen and you feel hungry. Under normal circumstances, a healthy person not on a diet will be eating balanced and regular meals, so these erratic hypoglycaemic swings won't happen. Blood glucose balance is maintained from one meal to the next.

But the low-calorie lifestyle of the dieter has already deliberately cut back on fuel supplies and the body isn't receiving enough sustenance to keep those appetite-controlling mechanisms in check. In addition to reducing food intake at mealtimes, dieters tend to miss breakfast, skip lunch and fill the gaps with coffee fixes, sugary snacks and late-night raids on the biscuit tin — action guaranteed to make hypoglycaemia much worse.

The cravings (most often for sweetness) happen because the body knows that very low blood glucose is a danger to life; if uncontrolled, leading to diabetes, coma and even death in extreme circumstances. All diabetics have suffered from hypoglycaemic attacks at one time or another but experience teaches them how to deal with the potential dangers. Taking something sweet is a very useful emergency antidote for serious hypos but is not to be recommended as a general rule. And yet some dieters resort to these extreme measures every day without realizing that they have become dependent upon a destructive addictive drug.

Once the blood glucose levels are pushed high again by that bar of chocolate or cream cake, the glucose-lowering hormone insulin is produced from the pancreas to bring the levels under control. But because, by now, the pancreas is so used to being overworked, it becomes 'trigger happy' and sends too much of the hormone into the blood. Glucose falls again very dramatically. You are right back where you started. A trigger-happy pancreas which is never allowed to rest will eventually take its own holiday by packing up altogether.

Not 'All In The Mind'

Any diet of poor quality (particularly a low-calorie one interspersed with sugar binges!) is likely to cause a disruption in brain chemistry, resulting in very real mental and emotional disturbance. You feel tetchy and tearful, your coordination is terrible, you drop things, bump into things and make mountains out of molehills. All reasons why hypoglycaemia is often mistaken for psychological problems; but the tangled thoughts have a physical cause. You are not neurotic and you're not going round the bend. Hypoglycaemia is far from being 'all in the mind'.

Hypoglycaemic First Aid

After a few weeks on the Food Combining Diet, your blood glucose should be back to normal and low blood sugar will be a thing of the past. The desire to eat between meals will diminish. In the meantime, however, it is absolutely vital to take your snacks seriously. You will see that the menus suggest midmorning snacks for the first two weeks. If, after this time, you don't feel any need to eat between meals, that's fine. But if you think you would continue to benefit from that extra piece of fruit or handful of seeds or nuts, then by all means keep them going for as long as you need to. Snacking is the most sensible way to maintain blood glucose balance and to prevent those terrible hypoglycaemic swings.

Following these tips should also help:

- Always have breakfast. Dr Hay recommended only a light fruit breakfast or no breakfast at all but, when you are starting out on the Hay Way, hypoglycaemia needs special handling. The menus include some hearty and sustaining breakfast meals but, if you are the kind of person who simply can't face food first thing in the morning, don't worry. Just have a light breakfast or a fruit snack as soon as you can manage it.
- If you are likely to be travelling or, for some other reason

unable to sit down to a proper meal, carry emergency supplies with you such as fresh fruit, sunflower or pumpkin seeds, unblanched almonds, a small container of fresh crudités or mixed dried fruit and nuts.

- Don't wait until you are sinking with hunger before you eat something.
- Don't go without food all day only to binge on a huge meal in the evening. The best philosophy for hypo sufferers is 'little and often'.
- Don't go to bed hungry. Snack on a small portion of yoghurt (protein) or a couple of rye crackers (starch) with a little butter. This will help to stabilize your blood glucose throughout the night. Waking up with night sweats is usually a sign that blood glucose levels are falling too far.
- Avoid 'quick-release' sugars such as sweet biscuits, cakes, pastries or chocolate — in fact, any food made from highly-refined white sugar or white flour. Excess amounts of cola, coffee, strong tea, fruit squashes, salt or alcohol can also contribute to hypo attacks.
- Stress will make matters worse. This is because the mechanism for raising the glucose levels in the blood is part of human evolution — a safety factor providing the body with enough instant energy to deal with life-endangering situations such as facing danger or for running away; the 'Fight or Flight Syndrome'. In today's stressful world, persistent mental and emotional overload has the same effect on the body's hormones as did the wild animal on the caveman!

Sweet Nothings

It is imperative that you avoid ordinary white or brown sugar. Nor would I recommend artificial sweeteners. The latest research tells us that diet foods, slimmers' meals and low-calorie drinks which contain artificial sweeteners are likely to make weight loss harder to achieve.[1] It seems that they can increase hunger pangs by disturbing blood glucose control and appetite;[2] their long term safety is also being called into question.[3,4]

Alternative Sweetenings (Starch)

If you have a sweet tooth, the thought of being without sugary foods can be a daunting one. However, as explained in the section on hypoglycaemia, the Food Combining Diet understands this and allows sweet treats and snacks.

For sweetening, you can use (in small quantities only):

Real maple syrup, blackstrap molasses, real Barbados sugar or honey. Choose organic, unblended honey for mixing with yoghurt, porridge, hot drinks etc. Avoid brands which say 'produce of more than one country' or 'blended' as this usually indicates that they have been heated, destroying goodness.

For baking, fructose is a better alternative than ordinary table sugar but is almost twice as sweet so take care with quantities. Other useful sweeteners are desiccated or creamed coconut and crystallized ginger.

All sweetenings are listed with starches. They are all acid-forming with the possible exception of blackstrap molasses which borders on neutral.

Sweet Treats (Starch)

After a few weeks on the Food Combining Diet, the risk of cravings and binges should be dwindling. However, if the thought of chocolate is burning a hole in your resolve, there are some healthier alternatives which may save your sanity. Treat all these confections as starch and use them in moderation only.

Carob is a Mediterranean native tree also known as St. John's Bread or Locust Bean since it is the 'locust' upon which John The Baptist is said to have survived his wanderings in the desert wilderness. The long pods of the carob tree are used to make a kind of vegetable chocolate which is available as a powder, 'chocolate' spread, as a covering for biscuits, raisins and cereal bars and to flavour drinks and desserts. In its raw state it contains very few calories and no fat although this status changes when it is mixed with other foods. Nutritionally, it is far superior to chocolate and contains no caffeine. Food combiners should list carob with starches because of its fructose (fruit sugar) content. It will not mix well with protein foods or with recipes which contain milk, so check label ingredients on carob products for milk content.

Natural liquorice sticks and sweets are available from health food stores. They should be eaten sparingly since an excess of liquorice will rob the body of potassium. Liquorice is a useful remedy for occasional constipation. Watch out for 'liquorice flavour' which may not be the real thing!

Sesame halva is an unusual sweet treat made with sesame seeds, honey and vanilla flavouring, sometimes with added almonds or dried fruit; an acquired taste but quite nutritious containing worthwhile amounts of iron, vitamin E and magnesium.

Unblanched almonds and raisins also make a good sweet-tasting snack but eat small amounts only.

Nearly all sweetenings have the potential to use up, destroy or hamper the absorption of vitamins, minerals and other nutrients.[5] *If you use added sugar of any kind, be sparing.*

Too Tired To Diet?

> 'God bless the inventor of sleep, the cloak that covers all men's thoughts, the food that cures all hunger . . . the balancing weight that levels the shepherd with the king and the simple with the wise.'
>
> *From* Don Quixote Pt II *by Miguel Cervantes (1547-1616)*

One of the most insufferable side effects of low-calorie dieting is the accompanying exhaustion. If you are not taking on board sufficient sustenance, there just aren't enough nutrients to manufacture energy. Lethargy looms large for every slimmer. But not with the Food Combining Diet — it's packed with power and vitality.

Rest, Relaxation and Sleep

Don't underestimate the recuperative powers of rest, relaxation and sleep. It can be a big mistake to rely solely upon exercise and diet alone in the pursuit of good health and well-being.

Much of the stress of modern living can come from the pressure of being always responsible for someone or something else — partner, boss, colleague, children, relatives, shopping, cooking, housework. Failing to take time and space for your own needs can result in both physical and emotional strain. However good your diet, it won't have the chance to do its best for you if you never take a break.

Simple changes which rest mind and body and give the system a change of scene can make an enormous difference. Visit the hairdresser or beauty salon, treat yourself to an aromatherapy massage or reflexology session, hide away for half an hour with a good book, take a deep bath, have a home facial, lie down and cat nap, sit quietly and listen to a relaxation cassette or radio play or go for a long walk.

Worry, anger, guilt and fear are destructive negative emotions which will do nothing for your long-term health and well-being. Share your cares and concerns with a confidant. Make a resolution to solve or surrender your anxieties rather than dwell on them. Nurture and nourish yourself for a change; and remember that it takes no more effort to be happy than it does to be miserable.

The Importance of
Detoxifying and Cleansing

―― ⫯ ――

Drink More Water

'Little drops of water, little grains of sand
Make the mighty ocean and the pleasant land
So the little minutes, humble though they be
Make the mighty ages of eternity.'
Little Things *by Julia Carney (1823-1908)*

It is rare that I meet a new patient who drinks enough water. Dieters, particularly, avoid drinking additional liquids in the mistaken belief that too much will increase their already bloated abdomen, tender breasts or swollen ankles. In fact, the opposite is true. Drinking *more* helps to reduce this uncomfortable inflammation. Too little fluid can lead to kidney and bladder problems, including urinary tract infections, and also encourages constipation and poor elimination of wastes.

The recommended *minimum* water intake per day is two pints (just over one litre) in addition to any tea, coffee and other fluids. Try to drink between meals and before meals but never with food — and never immediately afterwards (apart from the smallest mouthful which may be necessary in order to swallow any tablets you may be taking). Copious drinking with food simply makes the mixture too liquid and dilute, causing it to pass too rapidly through the system and preventing proper and complete digestion.

People who are unused to drinking water may baulk at what seems to be a large amount of fluid. Others say that they just don't feel thirsty and so forget to drink.

To increase your fluid intake, drink a small glass of water 10 or 15 minutes before each meal; also, keep a glass or cup of water near you and sip from it between meals. You'll be amazed at how often it needs refilling and how quickly you achieve your daily target. If you spend a lot of time behind the wheel, carry bottles of water with you. Most small water carriers will fit into door pockets or seat pouches.

A glass of tepid water (boiled and cooled, not taken from the hot tap) with a squeeze of fresh lemon juice first thing in the morning is an excellent cleanser and tonic. Lukewarm water is more helpful to the liver. The next best thing is water at room temperature but drinking very cold water is not recommended.

In addition to water, you can enjoy vegetable juices (steer clear of those which contain salt), fruit juices (always dilute them with water), fruit teas, herbal teas, grain-based coffee substitutes and dandelion coffee (a wonderful and natural diuretic). See 'Teas and Coffees'.

The use of filtered or distilled water is strongly recommended for drinking purposes, for filling the kettle and for cooking vegetables.

Never drink water from the hot tap or water which has been pre-softened.

Teas and Coffees

The Food Combining Diet does not expect you to give up tea or coffee. However, some people do indulge in rather large quantities of these beverages each day, often as a social habit rather than a real need. Try to limit yourself to three cups of tea or coffee (preferably less) each day. Use as little milk as possible — or, even better, no milk at all. Or try fresh lemon instead.

You could also experiment with herb teas but they can be an acquired taste — and you don't need to drink them unless you like them.

If you are trying to give up or cut down on coffee, experiment by mixing a quarter teaspoon of dandelion coffee (powder available from your health food store) with your usual coffee powder and, over a period of a few weeks, increase gradually on the dandelion and reduce the instant coffee.

If you are in the habit of having a cup of tea or coffee after lunch or dinner, try to leave an hour between the main course and any drink.

Detoxifying and Cleansing

After years of crash diets and see-saw weight loss and gain, helped along by a high intake of additive-laden processed food, any body is likely to become slow and sluggish. Energy and vitality can be forgotten feelings.

Our bodies tend to accumulate toxins (poisons) from many different sources including food additives, pesticide sprays, car exhaust fumes, medical drug residues and internal metabolic leftovers. If we are feeling under par and are carrying a little too much weight, the natural elimination of the wastes may be too slow for the body's own long-term good. Even in the best of circumstances, few people manage to escape pollution, exhaustion, stress, tension, anxiety, illness, overwork and rushed, hurried or missed meals; a typical scenario which can add up to only one thing: a toxic and overloaded system.

The Food Combining Diet not only introduces you to a new way of eating for good health and balanced weight control; it also incorporates a weekly detox diet which helps to clean the intestines, rest the digestion and restore sparkle and spirit.

Detox Diet

You will see from the Food Combining Diet menus that the 24 hours from Friday evening's supper through Saturday breakfast and Saturday lunch are made up only of fresh salads and fruits, no fat and no heavy protein. These clean alkaline-forming foods are easy on the digestion and help to flush out accumulated toxins from the bloodstream. Resting the digestion in this way also recharges the immune system and gives a tired body a real boost of energy.

If you find it inconvenient to follow the detox part of the programme on a Friday and Saturday, simply interchange these menus with some from another part of the week so that you follow the cleansing routine midweek instead.

The importance of drinking plenty of water throughout the Food Combining Diet cannot be over-emphasized.

The Importance of Good Circulation

Improving the circulation is a vital part of the cleansing and detoxifying process. Without efficient blood flow, oxygen and the microscopic nutrients from food cannot be moved efficiently around the body and wastes will not be properly discharged. An essential component of the detoxification mechanism is the R.E.S. (reticulo-endothelial system), a 'garbage truck' which collects foreign material, bacteria, dead tissue and other wastes from refuse outlets around the body and then drains them via the blood and lymph vessels into the general circulation to be eliminated. If the body has reached toxic overload, however, the system snarls up just like a fume-laden traffic jam. Nothing moves and the pollution levels rise higher and higher. The ultimate consequence of this build-up is 'dis'-ease in its many forms often beginning with chronic fatigue, poor weight control, a compromised immune system and susceptibility to viral and bacterial invasion.

A major stepping stone in the healing process is to improve the functioning of the circulatory systems so that nutrients are delivered to where they are needed and the junk is taken away. Good circulation is vital to efficient lymph drainage and R.E.S. function which simply cannot work if the blood isn't pumping properly.

Skin Brushing

To speed lymph drainage, remove dead skin cells, improve circulation and enhance the whole detoxification process, skin brushing or loofah brushing is also recommended. Although the natural bristle skin brush is normally used dry – before bathing – this may not suit some ultra-sensitive skins. An effective alternative is a loofah, natural sponge or rough flannel face cloth massaged over wet skin. Using firm stroking movements, cover as much of the body as you can reach but pay particular attention to the neck, chest, under and inner arms, abdomen and legs, especially the inner thighs and backs of the knees.

The Healing Crisis

When you first begin, you may experience something which naturopaths call 'a healing crisis'. As the body throws off unwanted substances, its main elimination apparatus (bowel, lungs, liver, kidneys and bladder, skin, blood, lymph, and the female menstrual flow) is working overtime. Headaches, slight nausea, diarrhoea, heavier than usual periods, skin irritation, even a cold are signs that the detoxification process is under way. Taking painkillers, antacids or over-the-counter cold remedies may serve only to drive the toxins back into the liver and bloodstream, thereby reversing the beneficial elimination process.

If you are affected by a healing crisis, here's what to do:

1. Stop working.
2. Become unavailable!
3. Have a deep, warm and soothing bath perhaps with some lavender and marjoram essential oils.
4. Go to bed for 24 hours and rest.
5. Drink plenty of water.
6. Take 1 gram of buffered vitamin C every 3 hours for 3 or 4 days.

Constipation is a common problem for dieters, especially those who don't take on board enough fibre, water or nutrients. If constipation is a problem for you, try these tips:

• Include plenty of *cold pressed oils* in the diet. A tablespoon or two each day of extra virgin olive oil is an excellent bowel lubricant.
• Check out the *fibre* in your present diet. The Food Combining Diet has a wealth of gentle and beneficial fibre in the form of fruits, vegetables, wholegrains, salads, seeds and nuts. *Dried figs* are particularly helpful.
• *Linseeds* are especially good for stubborn constipation. They are tiny golden seeds rich in essential fatty acids. Always buy them in sealed packets — never loose — and keep them in the fridge. Eat them on their own, mixed with yoghurt or sprinkled onto porridge or salads. One tablespoon daily is usually sufficient to persuade things to happen!
• Extra fibre in the diet demands additional fluids so make sure you have plenty of *water and juices*.

- *Abdominal massage* is a wonderfully relaxing way to ease a tense colon. Use olive oil or olive oil cream and massage gently but firmly with the pads of the fingers over the whole of the abdomen, using a firm circular action and paying particular attention to the area which covers the large bowel.

- *Deep breathing exercises* really do help a difficult bowel. Shallow breathing allows toxins to build up in the bloodstream, reduces the efficiency of nutrient transport and denies the body its life-sustaining oxygen supply. If the tissues are not receiving sufficient oxygen, cells can become 'rigid' and muscles tense. If muscles are not relaxed, the movement of wastes through the bowel, controlled by a muscular squeezing action called peristalsis, slows down or stops altogether. Faeces accumulate and become impacted, making elimination more and more difficult.

    Filling the lungs and moving the diaphragm and abdominal muscles with each breath stimulates detoxification, improves muscle tone and generally revives inactive internal workings. Deep breathing also relaxes and de-stresses an overactive mind.

Regular exercise also plays a vital role in detoxification. See page 48 for more information on exercise.

Friendly Bacteria

A major reason for persistent and resistant constipation can be a disturbance in the balance and ratio of friendly to unfriendly bacteria in the gut. The gastrointestinal tract plays host to a vast quantity of active micro-organisms totalling several pounds in weight. When elimination is poor, stale faecal matter builds up inside the colon, putrefies (goes off!) and makes a rather nasty, smelly food supply for bacteria, yeast and other beasties. These little horrors are only too happy to digest your badly digested leftovers but, when they've eaten their fill, what they throw out as wastes are lots of different toxins which delight in upsetting the friendly flora. Pork and beef are two of the foods most likely to putrefy and sustain these bubble blowing and bloating bugs.

When the build up of toxicity reaches overload, the junk is allowed to seep into the bloodstream, just like poisonous industrial waste trickles undetected into rivers and streams. No-one notices until the fish begin to die. In the same way, whilst you may have noticed the odd feeling of unwellness, it can take years of increasing imbalances within the human body before the clear and obvious symptoms of disease manifest themselves.

There are many things in the modern external environment which are able to cause or aggravate this imbalance, not least the overuse of antibiotics either via doctors' prescriptions or in animal feedstuffs. Broad-spectrum antibiotics are blind. They fire off their bacteria-killing bullets indiscriminately and don't stop to distinguish between the beneficial and non-beneficial bacteria.

But it's not all bad news. Where good health is maintained, the 'good' keep the 'bad' under control and this terrifying scenario of destruction and illness is prevented.

Probiotic Paratroopers

One of the simplest and safest ways of restoring balance is to replace the good bacteria in the form of probiotic (pro-life) supplements and food which contains friendly flora such as live yoghurt.

Probiotic powders contain beneficial bacteria such as *Lactobacillus acidophilus* and *Bifidus*, natural inhabitants of the gut, able to take control of the proliferating enemy. Since it has often taken many years to destroy the favourable habitat of the intestines, it can take several months to restore the balance. Supplementation is therefore usually recommended over a period of six to twelve months accompanied by a healthy diet.

Live yoghurt can be enormously helpful in hastening improvements, but check to make sure the yoghurt you are buying contains the right kind of *Lactobacillus acidophilus* bacteria. If it's in there, the label should tell you so.

If you are concerned about your health or are undergoing medical treatment, please check with your doctor and dietitian before starting any diet. If your constipation is not responding to dietary changes or if you have noticed any alterations in bowel habit recently, i.e. swelling, pain, bleeding, stools which are darker than usual or difficult to flush away, please do consult your doctor without delay.

The Importance of Regular Exercise

For many people, the thought of exercise can conjure up as many negatives as a deprivation diet. Boring, time-consuming, painful, exhausting, a complete waste of effort.

But it doesn't need to be. The positive profits of balanced and habitual movement are enormous. Research shows that a sensible level of regular exercise can have many health benefits, such as reduced blood pressure,[1,2,3] improved oxygen uptake,[4] better muscle tone and lean body mass,[5] reduced risk of a difficult pregnancy and labour,[6] enhanced immune function, better digestion, improved quality of life and less degenerative disease.[7] Females who take regular exercise are at much less risk of osteoporosis.[8] Exercise also improves mood, reduces anxiety and depression and dissolves negative stress.[9,10] Another positive point is that adding exercise to a sensible diet can almost double the percentage of body fat lost.[11]

Work Out With Care

As with everything else in life, exercise taken to excess has a detrimental effect upon the body. Fitness freaks who work out to extremes are not exercising but indulging in strenuous over-exertion. Overdoing things can damage the skeletal frame, reduce resistance to infection, cause nutrient loss and disturb hormone imbalance.[12] There is no need to suffer hours of burnout aerobics or run a marathon every day to stay fit and healthy. Swimming, rebounding (mini-trampolining), gentle (low impact) aerobics, keep fit classes, dancing, yoga, moderate weight training, stretching and deep breathing are all beneficial types of exercise. Rebounding for ten minutes can be as effective as half an hour pounding the tarmac, without the weather problems, pollution or need for specialist clothing; and you don't need high ceilings.

And the benefits of brisk walking should not be dismissed. In a study carried out by the Cooper Institute for Aerobics Research, women participants showed improved oxygen uptake and cardiovascular performance even when walking at a steady pace. In other words, there are still benefits to be had from exercise that is not particularly vigorous.[13] Aim to exercise for 15 to 20 minutes every day or 40 minutes two or three times a week.

If you are new to any exercise programme, ask for specialist assistance from a qualified fitness expert, aerobics teacher, swimming coach or gym instructor. If you have an existing health problem and are receiving medication, check first with your practitioner before embarking on any new fitness activity.

Don't Eschew Chewing

One type of exercise rarely mentioned is that of chewing. Proper mastication helps to keep gums, teeth and jaw strong and healthy but also improves digestion which, in turn, encourages efficient metabolism.

An early proponent of nutritional therapy was an American called Horace Fletcher (1849–1919) who proved that 'industrious munching' helps to increase weight loss. Proper mastication, he demonstrated, satisfies a hearty appetite. Food should be reduced by the teeth and saliva to a pulp before swallowing. In his own case, Horace lost over 40 pounds (3 stones) in just a few months by increasing chewing activity.

To Help Improve Your Digestion

'Bad men live to eat and drink, whereas good men eat and drink in order to live.'

Socrates (469–399 BC)
Greek philosopher

- Eat when you are hungry. Don't be forced into food just because the clock says it is time to eat. Conversely, don't put up with emptiness or hunger pangs.
- Always have breakfast.
- Avoid large amounts of fluid with meals.
- Drink plenty of filtered water between meals. Chlorine and aluminium in tap water do seem to aggravate digestive disorders in some people.
- Keep all fruits and fruit juices away from main meals whenever possible. Don't gulp them or drink them 'on the move'. Sip and savour them.
- Wash all fruits and vegetables thoroughly before using.

Avoid eating fruit skins unless you know they are unsprayed.

- Some digestion begins in the mouth, so chew all food really thoroughly, particularly nuts, seeds, beans and wholegrains. If you have dental problems and chewing is difficult for you, try chopping, liquidizing and grating food.
- Don't eat foods which are very hot or very cold.
- Reduce your intake of coffee, tea and cola.
- Try to avoid convenience and take-away foods and those which contain refined sugar, refined flour, high levels of salt or stimulating spices i.e. chilli, curry etc.
- Keep bread and other wheat products to a minimum.
- Try to avoid aluminium. Don't use aluminium pans or allow foil to touch food. Steer clear of ordinary brand toothpastes, some of which contain aluminium; change to a natural herbal or mineral toothpaste. Dried milk powders and dried soups may include aluminium silicate as an anti-caking agent. Many prescribed medicines, particularly those used to treat over-acidity, also contain aluminium.
- After a few weeks of proper food combining, indigestion should be a thing of the past. If, however, you have to use an indigestion remedy in an emergency, choose a natural herbal one made from something like meadowsweet and medicinal charcoal rather than proprietary medicines which are often high in aluminium.
- Avoid rich food and keep meals simple.
- Allow time between courses.
- Always sit for at least ten minutes after eating. Don't rush around or take vigorous exercise for at least one hour after a meal.
- An interval of approximately 4 hours should elapse between protein meals and starch meals.
- The regular reheating of meals is not recommended since it impairs flavour, disturbs digestion and destroys nutrients. In addition, stored cooked food — even when kept in a refrigerator — can breed bacteria. If reheating is unavoidable,

make sure that the food is hot right through (not just around the edges) before serving. Food should never be reheated more than once.

- Eating a small quantity of raw salad before a cooked meal with 15 minutes or so between courses will further assist the digestive process.
- Never eat when overtired, anxious or stressed.
- DON'T MIX FOODS THAT FIGHT.

Getting the Chemistry Right

❦

'Dis-moi ce que tu manges et je te dirai ce que tu es.'
'Tell me what you eat and I will tell you what you are.'
Anthelme Brillat-Savarin (1755-1826)
French politician and gourmet

This is no boring science lesson but an exciting illustration of how food can directly affect the way you look and the way you feel. Understand the importance of balancing blood chemistry and you are a step nearer to restoring your sparkle and spirit — and to shedding that excess weight.

Everything we eat has either an ACID-FORMING or ALKALINE-FORMING effect upon our bodies and one of the most vital doctrines of the Hay Way is to achieve the optimum balance between these two headings. But there is no need to worry about this ratio.

The Food Combining Diet Menus have been designed to guide you; they are high in healthy alkaline-forming fresh fruits, salads and vegetables, low in fat and low in acid-forming proteins and added sugars.

It can seem contrary that a food which is 'acidic' before being eaten, such as grapefruit for example, should become 'alkaline-forming' once it has been dealt with by the body. But this is exactly what happens.

Whether or not a food is acid-forming or alkaline-forming is determined by the mineral 'ash' which remains after food has been digested, absorbed and metabolized.

Alkaline-forming salads, fruits and vegetables leave valuable residues of such minerals as calcium, magnesium and potassium. Acid-forming meals (meat, fish and most grains, pulses and nuts, for example), deposit chlorine, sulphur and phosphorus in the bloodstream. To maintain tiptop health, we all need to choose foods from both groups but, at the same time, heed Dr Hay's warning that too many acid-forming foods can create 'internal pollution', 'self-poisoning' and 'acid-autotoxicosis'. Don't we all know an over-stressed, grey-faced, paunch-over-trouser-belt business executive prone to a sour stomach, hangover headaches, pungent sweat and grouchy insensitivity? I have witnessed this acid state of affairs many times in patients whose diets consisted originally and predominantly of toast and coffee breakfasts, alcohol lunches and lots of late-in-the-evening dinners heavy with meat and rich sauces! The remarkable improvement in their general health and well-being when they became food combining converts is wonderful to see.

Apart from helping to restore normal bodyweight, foods of the alkaline-forming persuasion have many other talents. Clinical experience would seem to suggest that the beneficial increase in alkalinity in the body's tissues can help to reduce addictions and cravings. Good for smokers and chocoholics alike!

Acid/Alkaline-Forming Foods

Calming, cleansing and nourishing, the 'alkalines' are rich in vitamins, minerals and fibre, low in sugar and low in fat.

As Celia Wright points out in her book *The Wright Diet*, increasing the body's vital alkaline reserve will make you feel 'very good, good in body, good in mind' whereas an over-acid state can leave you resembling a 'cross rat that just fell out the wrong side of bed'.

Keep Things Simple

When I first set foot on the Hay Way, I followed one very general rule during the early stages which might help you as you begin.

> Remember that:
>   Most fruits and vegetables are alkaline-forming
>   Most proteins and starches are acid-forming
> or, put another way:
>   Foods which are digested and absorbed quickly by the body
>   (fruits and vegetables) tend to be alkaline-forming
>   Foods which take longer to digest (proteins and starches) tend
>   to be acid-forming.

There are, of course, a few exceptions which you will learn quickly and easily from the charts and lists provided.

Throughout the book:
  Alkaline-forming foods are marked with a plus sign: +
  Acid-forming foods are marked with a minus sign: −
  'N' indicates foods which are neither acid-forming nor alkaline-forming.

But don't be too concerned about remembering these at the outset. Let the Food Combining Diet Menus guide you for the first month.

When you plan your own menus, daily balance will be maintained by having:

One completely alkaline-forming meal
One starch-based meal
One protein-based meal

Example 1:
An alkaline-forming fruit breakfast
A starch-based lunch of brown rice and salad
A protein supper of fresh fish (or tofu with mushrooms) with
   stir-fried or steamed vegetables.

Example 2:
A starch-based breakfast of muesli or porridge
A protein lunch of free-range chicken or a cheese dish with
   vegetables or salad
An alkaline-forming supper of mixed salad.

Note: Vegetarians and vegans will find a wonderful selection of
recipes — including such gems as a starch-free pie crust — in
Jackie Le Tissier's book *Food Combining For Vegetarians*.

Rest and Relax

Remember that smoking, alcohol, lack of sleep, excessive stress,
overwork, exhaustion, worry and negative thoughts such as fear
are all *acid-forming*.

Food Groups
Explained — Proteins

❧

Protein foods are all kinds of cheese, yoghurt, milk, eggs, all kinds of meat, all kinds of fish and soya products.

Cheeses (Acid-Forming/Protein)

All cheeses are classed as protein foods. So hard farmhouse cheeses, goat's cheese, cottage cheese, Greek Feta, French Brie, Camembert and so on will mix happily with other protein foods, vegetables and salads but not with starch. Feta cheese is very salty but the salt can be reduced by soaking the cheese in water overnight.

In some food combining books, *dairy cream cheese* is listed as an exception to the rule, being high in fat with a relatively low protein content and, as such, is classed as (neutral) fat, compatible with starches. This may only apply in the U.K., however, and not to American, Australian or some European cream cheeses which can have a much higher protein content.

Most cream cheese sold from U.K. stores is made with super double cream and contains around 45 per cent fat but only 3 per cent protein. To avoid confusion and incompatibility, my advice would be to treat all cheeses as proteins but to accept that U.K. cream cheese may be suitable, occasionally, for use with starches — say as a jacket potato topping, for example.

There is a particular distinction between *dairy cream cheese* and the similar-in-appearance *soft cheese* so check with your grocer or supermarket before you buy.

Full fat soft cheese is usually made with skimmed milk and some double cream. It is classed as a protein.

Low fat soft cheese is made with buttermilk and a lactic acid culture not dissimilar to that used for yoghurt making. It has a correspondingly lower fat content but is classified as protein.

Good quality low fat soft cheese is a healthy alternative to cottage cheese which contains no culture and can be high in salt. Always read product labels, however. Some low fat cheeses, especially prepackaged ones, may contain lots of additives.

It can be a mistake to rely too heavily on cheese as a meat substitute; fat intake can creep up stealthily without you even realizing it. When using hard cheeses for protein dishes, choose the stronger-tasting farmhouse varieties; you need less. Avoid all processed, smoked and coloured cheeses.

Yoghurt (Alkaline-Forming/Protein)

Yoghurt is an excellent source of good quality protein, calcium, potassium and magnesium. It also contains some B vitamins, zinc and vitamin A (less vitamin A in the low fat varieties). 'Yoghurt' is an anglicized version of a Turkish word meaning 'fermented milk'.

Since the discovery that the bacteria cultures used in yoghurt making may be beneficial to our health, supermarket shelves have been filling up with greater and grander varieties of 'live', 'lacto' and 'bio' products. Here's how to tell the difference:

All standard ordinary yoghurts are made with pasteurized full fat cow's milk; low fat yoghurts with skimmed milk. Cultures of *Streptococcus lactus* and *Streptococcus thermophilus* are then added. The mixtures are incubated in large tanks and stirred to make them into a thick liquid. During manufacture, the milk sugar (lactose) is broken down into lactic acid by the yoghurt culture which coagulates the milk and makes it easier to digest.

The firmer set yoghurts go through an identical process to the more liquid yoghurts but are allowed to incubate and set in the pot rather than in tanks and are not stirred. Setting agents are sometimes used.

Bio yoghurts undergo the same process and can be set or liquid. The difference lies in the choice of culture — usually *Lactobacillus acidophilus* — considered more beneficial because it is a natural inhabitant of the human gut. Another culture — called *Lactobacillus bulgaricus* — is used less frequently because it gives yoghurt a sharper, tart flavour — not so popular.

There are a few yoghurts on the market which are heat-treated by sterilization and so no longer contain their original culture. These should be classed as extremely acid-forming and are not recommended.

Read the labels and look out for those which contain the beneficial cultures — or make your own with a good starter culture. Try to avoid flavoured and fruit yoghurts; they can be very high in sugar and sweeteners and may not contain real fruit. For example, 'blackcurrant flavoured' means it is flavoured with real blackcurrants but 'blackcurrant flavour' may mean artificial or nature-identical additives.

Remember that, from the food combining point of view, cultured yoghurts are healthily alkaline-forming. All yoghurts should be refrigerated and consumed before the Use-by date.

Milk (Acid-Forming/Protein if Pasteurized; Alkaline-Forming/Protein if Raw, Unpasteurized)

Milk is a complete protein. In its raw state, milk is alkaline-forming but becomes increasingly acid-forming the more it is heat treated. This means that nearly all the readily available bottled and cartoned milks are acid-forming because they have been pasteurized or sterilized.

Milk does not mix well with other foods. Mammalian milks are species specific – in other words, they suit the species for which they were intended. Cow's milk is extremely suitable for calves. Infant humans thrive on human breast milk but their digestive systems are not designed to continue consuming pasteurized cow's milk into adulthood. Cow's milk mixed with other foods is particularly difficult for the human digestion to handle and will fight with both starches and proteins. If you do use milk, don't combine it with other foods except in the minutest quantities.[1] And bear in mind that drug, hormone and pesticide residues do pass from the feed into the milk supply.

What About Calcium?

Don't be concerned that, if you cut your milk intake, you will be deficient in calcium. Whilst it is true that cow's milk contains ample amounts, it is certainly not the only calcium source, this mineral being available from many foods. Diets which are too high in protein will affect calcium levels whilst absorption of calcium from cow's milk is generally poor where there are enzyme and stomach acid deficiencies – both extremely common in adults and a particular problem for the elderly.[2,3,4] You'll find calcium in yoghurt (easier to digest than milk), eggs, cheese, canned salmon and sardines, wholegrains including oats, corn and brown rice, root vegetables, winter cabbage, broccoli, watercress and fresh fish. But this is not an exhaustive list; calcium is available in smaller amounts in a wide range of foods. Tofu (soya bean curd), pulses and nuts also contain calcium but should be eaten in strict moderation only.

· Raw or 'Green' Milk (Alkaline-Forming/Protein)

Unprocessed organic raw milk (i.e. 'green' or unpasteurized) is alkaline-forming because it hasn't been heat treated. If you use raw milk, make sure that it comes from a recognized and reliable supplier.

Goat's and Sheep's Milk (Acid-Forming/Protein if Pasteurized; Alkaline-Forming/Protein if Raw, Unpasteurized)

Those with cow's milk intolerance may find that they are able to drink goat's or sheep's milk instead. Sometimes dismissed as strong-smelling, these milks will only give off an unpleasant odour if they are not fresh. Both are convenient in that they freeze well but, once thawed, should be used within 48 hours. Both are richer than cow's milk and can be diluted with 20 per cent (filtered) water if required. Again, use in strict moderation and do not mix with other foods except in the minutest quantities.

Soya Milk (Acid-Forming/Protein)

Soya 'milk' — more properly 'soya drink' — is not a milk but a white liquid made from soya beans. It can provide a useful milk substitute but these following points should be borne in mind:

1. Firstly, soya drink is a manufactured, processed food and so, therefore, would not concur with Dr. Hay's teachings.
2. Secondly, the protein molecules in soya drink are extremely large — larger than those in cow's milk — putting yet more strain on the digestive system.

3. Thirdly, whilst soya drinks are usually fortified with vitamins and minerals in an attempt to equal cow's milk's nutrient status, the calcium is unlikely to be well absorbed.

If you use it, keep to small quantities. For food combining purposes, it should be treated as an acid-forming protein food along with other soya products — tofu, tempeh, miso, soya flour etc.

Eggs (Acid-Forming/Protein)

Eggs have been much maligned in recent years for their cholesterol content. Anyone suspected of having coronary heart disease was warned to avoid eggs for this reason. Research has now shown, however, that the cholesterol in food has little, if any, effect upon the levels of cholesterol in blood.[5]

In some food combining books, egg yolk is listed under fats and egg white under protein, indicating that it would be acceptable to mix egg yolks with starches. But egg yolks, in fact, are rich in protein; mixing egg yolks with starchy foods creates mucus and hampers digestion. Treat yolks *and* whites of egg as proteins.

Always use true free-range eggs. Those from battery-reared hens may contain artificial colours and additives. Bear in mind that the terms 'farm fresh' and 'barn eggs' do not signify free range. Boil, scramble, poach or bake eggs. Never fry them.

Fish (Acid-Forming/Protein)

Fish provides a nourishing low-fat protein alternative to meat and cheese. Studies have demonstrated the benefits of fish, especially the oily kind, in reducing heart disease risk.[6,7] Fish is also rich in the fat-soluble vitamins A and D.

Always buy really fresh fish and use it within 24 hours. A strong fishy smell usually indicates that it is not fresh. Some commercially frozen fish is sprayed with chemicals (the labelling doesn't have to tell you this!) so if you find it convenient to keep fish in your freezer, buy it fresh and freeze it yourself. Salted and smoked fish are not recommended.

Meat (Acid-Forming/Protein)

No factory-farmed beef or pork, battery-raised poultry or their by-products i.e. beefburgers, ham, bacon, pork pies, chicken pies, sausages etc. are recommended on the Food Combining Diet. Many are unsuitable from a food combining point of view since mixed and minced meat products may also contain starch in the form of breadcrumbs, flour and pastry. They are often high in fat and rich in additives too.

Having studied these foods — and witnessed symptoms caused by their detrimental effects — I have yet to be convinced that they are healthy. There are simply too many reports of unfit meat, drug residues, salmonella, illegal steroid use, B.S.E. and the appalling treatment suffered by factory-farmed animals to encourage me to think otherwise.[8,9,10] Who wants mad cows for lunch or sad hens for supper, anyway?

An additional problem is the length of time it takes for meat to pass through the long and twisted workings of the human gut; it should be just a few hours but, commonly, takes several days during which time it putrefies and discharges toxins into the bloodstream. Bad breath, body odour, excessive sweating, poor skin, foul-smelling stools and pungent feet are common symptoms.

In the Food Combining Diet, the majority of meals are meat-free. Only occasional free-range lamb and free-range poultry are included. When choosing meat, ask your butcher or meat counter if organically-reared products are available. Sometimes, prices for organic meat are a little higher but the costs tend to average out since you will be eating less meat overall.

Food Groups
Explained — Starches

───────────── ❧ ─────────────

Starches, sometimes also referred to as carbohydrates, include oats, rye, rice, barley, buckwheat, millet, pasta, all kinds of flour (except soya) and any food made from grain-based products, including bread, biscuits and crackers. 'Complex carbohydrates' (polysaccharides) is the term used to mean the wholegrain version i.e. whole oats, oat cakes, brown rice, wholewheat pasta, wholegrain bread, whole rye biscuits etc. The Food Combining Diet recommends wholegrains. With the exception of alkaline-forming millet, all grains are acid-forming.

Because of their high concentrations of carbohydrates (in the form of sugars), very sweet fruits and some dried fruits also come under the heading of starch.

A Word About Wheat Bran

'Breakfast foods are dusty and cold', wrote Ogden Nash and, indeed, many people still plough dutifully through masses of brown string and sawdust every day in the interests of a contented colon.

Wheat bran really lives up to the 'roughage' tag. Harsh, rough and irritating to the sensitive colon wall, it is a common culprit in food intolerance *and* in bowel disorders.

One of Dr Hay's abiding beliefs was that 'death begins in the colon' and that proper elimination and a healthy bowel are important steps to improving health. But eliminating with a poor quality or damaging fibre can inflict unnecessary suffering on an already sensitive gut.

The Food Combining Diet recommends avoiding wheat bran and wheat-based cereals, preferring instead the more gentle wholegrains such as oat-based home-made muesli and oat bran porridge and brown rice.

Constipation is unlikely to be a problem when you have been Food Combining for a few weeks. (See pages 42–48 which explain the importance of proper elimination, cleansing and detoxification.)

Bread (Acid-Forming/Starch)

Good quality bread can provide a healthy amount of daily fibre together with valuable nutrients such as iron, potassium, magnesium, zinc and B vitamins. Before the days of supermarkets and convenience foods, bread was produced either by the local baker or at home with only the most basic of ingredients – flour, yeast, water and salt. Freshly baked every day, stale leftovers were usually relegated to bread crumbs or bird food.

Not so now. Most bread is made by an industrial method which uses double the amount of yeast and rapid fermentation with loaves rising in a few minutes instead of a few hours. 'Improvers' help to retain softness so that a loaf can appear to be fresh many days after purchase. Additives may include such delights as monoacetyltartaric acid and diacetyltartaric acid esters, hydrogenated vegetable oils, chlorine dioxide, azodi-carbonamide, potassium bromate and disodium dihydrogen diphosphate. Unwrapped breads are exempt from labelling but may still contain several additives including colourings.

Some 'brown' breads are just white breads disguised with artificial caramel. Cushion-like sponginess is usually a sign that the bread contains additional yeast and extra gluten — a sticky protein found in grains which is also a common allergen. Chronic fatigue and lethargy are common symptoms in people sensitive to gluten, wheat and yeast.

Bread can aggravate mucus production. Modern 'mega-processed' varieties of bread are extremely mucus-forming and should, therefore, be used with caution by anyone who suffers with sinus problems, catarrh, digestive or bowel disorders. They are not recommended on the Food Combining Diet. Toasting bread destroys some of the B vitamins but also lessens the mucus-forming properties.

If you enjoy bread but don't have the time or the inclination to make your own, there are still plenty of alternatives to the squashy supermarket varieties. You could try the traditional yeast-free wholemeal soda breads, wholewheat pittas and old-fashioned wholegrain loaves made with organic stoneground flours. Dark or black rye (also called Pumpernickel and Schinkenbrot) is an excellent option for those who cannot tolerate wheat products. Dark rye has a close, heavy texture and a 'sourdough' flavour. Usually vacuum-wrapped and additive-free, it has a long shelf life and freezes well but should be used up within a few days once opened.

Breakfast Cereals (Acid-Forming/Starch)

Most pre-packed mueslis or mixed cereals are a poor protein/starch combination and the majority are wheat-based with very high sugar and salt. The famous brown string variety, for example, contains nearly 20 per cent (one-fifth) sugar and high levels of salt.

The Food Combining Diet recommends using home-made muesli (so that you can control the quality and quantity of the ingredients — the recipe is in the Menus section) and oat porridge. Both these breakfasts are sustaining and filling, providing stacks of nourishment and good levels of dietary fibre. Since the amount of oatmeal in the muesli recipe is so very small, it is quite acceptable to mix it with the apple and apple juice — a combination which would not be recommended if there was a larger starch content.

Wheatgerm and Oatgerm

Wheatgerm is made up of the small creamy-coloured flakes which are removed during the milling of white flour. In its fresh state, it contains plenty of minerals and is a good fibre source. Unfortunately, however, wheatgerm turns rancid very quickly and also can be a problem for those with an allergy to wheat products. I have not recommended it on the Food Combining Diet but, if you do use it, buy only small amounts at a time in a sealed container which shows a clear use-by date. Never buy loose wheatgerm: exposure to air, light and warmth will have already triggered deterioration.

If you are wheat-sensitive, oatgerm is a good alternative and is available from selected health food stores and delicatessens. Whichever you choose, store them in airtight containers in the refrigerator.

Pasta (Acid–Forming/Starch)

This highly nutritious food has always received a bad press because of its calorie content. But pasta is packed with nutrients and, since it is so filling, only small portions are required.

Pasta is the generic name for a multitude of different shapes made from a basic mixture of flour and water. Most pasta is made from durum semolina which takes longer to digest than the more common bread wheats but does not seem to cause the violent allergic reactions associated with bread and wheat cereals. In other words, whilst some people are intolerant of all wheat products, others find that pasta is acceptable even when bread may cause them digestive discomfort. Rice and corn pasta are available from some health food stores and delicatessens.

Wholemeal pasta provides a valuable source of magnesium, iron, potassium, zinc, B vitamins and dietary fibre. Serving pasta with fresh salads or vegetables will help to enhance the absorption of nutrients, particularly the iron.

Brown Rice (Acid-Forming/Starch)

Wholegrain rice is rich in magnesium, iron and B vitamins, provides a useful mixture of soluble and insoluble dietary fibre and is gluten-free. Rice is extremely versatile and comes in many different varieties; aromatic, brown, wild, basmati and jasmine to name only a few. It also provides the base for a range of food products including rice cakes, crackers, noodles, pasta, flakes, cereals, bran and flour. It takes 300 gallons of water to grow one pound (16 ounces/450 grams) of rice.

One cup of raw dry rice will make 3 cups when cooked. To test for readiness, press a few grains between finger and thumb. They should separate cleanly without leaving any hard core. Remember that B vitamins will be lost if the rice is overboiled.

Jacket Potatoes (Alkaline-Forming/Starch)

The humble spud is believed to originate from Chile. Called *pappas* by the South American Indians and *batata* by the Spaniards, it was brought to Spain and Portugal by explorers in the early 1500s. Sir Francis Drake is accredited with its original discovery and its introduction to England in 1577 where 'batata' became 'potato'. Sir Walter Ralegh took seed potatoes to Ireland in 1585.

A staple, nutritious and filling starch, jacket potatoes provide potassium, iron, C and B vitamins and, when cooked, will contain more nutrients than boiled potatoes which lose much goodness into the cooking water. Most commercially-grown potatoes are dowsed with chemicals including anti-sprouting sprays so if organic, unsprayed potatoes are not available, don't eat the skins! When preparing potatoes, always remove any eyes or green parts.

Food Groups Explained — Neutral Foods

❧

Note: Neutral foods can be acid- or alkaline-forming. The term 'neutral' merely indicates that they mix with either proteins or starches.

Be Adventurous With Vegetables

Vegetables figure prominently in the Food Combining Diet. And for good reason. Rich in vitamins and minerals, low in calories, low in fat, high in fibre and unprocessed, these foods provide the body with top class nourishment. Vegetables and saladings are alkaline-forming. They combine well with each other and with either starches or proteins.

HEALTH NOTE: PESTICIDE SPRAYS

It is almost impossible these days to obtain unsprayed, organic fruit and vegetables. In season, home-grown produce is less likely to have been saturated with fungicides and pesticides but don't be afraid to ask plenty of questions of your supplier.

A great deal of the fruit and vegetables sold in the U.K. is imported and, currently, we have no way of knowing which sprays are used and to what density or frequency. Although many dietitians advise that fruit skins should be eaten for their beneficial fibre, I tend to the view that we are better off without too many chemicals. For this reason, I advise my own patients to discard the peel from non-organic fruits, particularly apples and pears. In any event, all produce should be washed extremely thoroughly and then wiped or blotted with kitchen paper or a cotton cloth before preparation. Although some sprays are bound to penetrate the flesh, you would be amazed at how much dirt, bacteria and undesirable toxicity can be removed by thorough cleaning. Further information on sources of organic produce appear at the back of the book.

A Note About Nuts and Seeds

Nuts

Treat all nuts as acid-forming with the exception of almonds and brazils.

Nuts are an extremely concentrated food and should be eaten in small amounts only. They are best combined with vegetables and salads but small quantities could be added to protein or starch dishes. Check the Food Lists (at the back of the book) for compatibility.

Due to their rich content of unsaturated oils, nuts can become rancid very easily once shelled. Wherever possible, buy them in the shells. Shelled nuts should be absolutely fresh, unbroken and sold in sealed bags marked clearly with a use-by date. Never buy loose nuts (i.e. from 'serve yourself' hoppers) or those displayed on open counters in bright daylight.

Always eat nuts slowly, chewing them as thoroughly as possible before swallowing.

Seeds

Most edible seeds are rich sources of vitamins, minerals and essential fatty acids. For the Food Combining Diet, treat seeds as alkaline-forming. They combine acceptably with both starches or proteins.

The special unsaturated oils in seeds are as susceptible to

rancidity as the oils which are made from them, so proper use and storage is essential. Buy only sealed dated packets, never loose, and store in an airtight container in the refrigerator. Avoid roasted seeds.

Generally, seeds are gentle on the digestion and excellent for a sluggish bowel but, if you do find them at all indigestible, try grinding them in a food processor or coffee grinder before serving.

Fats and Oils

Fats and oils are neutral in that they are neither acid- nor alkaline-forming. You will see from the Menus and from the Food Lists on pages 159–170, that only certain fats and oils are recommended.

For Cooking

For cooking and stir-frying, use small amounts of butter or extra virgin olive oil, rather than other kinds of fats and oils. Take care not to heat these to very high temperatures (i.e. smoking heat) as this not only impairs digestibility but also distorts the chemical structure of the oil or fat, making it less healthy.

For Spreading

If you need a spreading fat for bread, biscuits or crackers, use real butter and avoid completely any polyunsaturated or low-fat spreads which are made from hydrogenated vegetable oils. Most supermarket spreading fats are made this way so check the labels.

For many years now, polyunsaturates have been synonymous with reducing heart disease. Many of us leapt dutifully on to the polyunsaturated bandwagon and felt confident that we were eating healthily.

The polyunsaturates with which we are most familiar are those sold as spreadable 'margarines'. But mounting evidence suggests that these may not be so good for us after all.[1] Natural polyunsaturates are those oils, naturally liquid at room temperature, which are extracted from vegetables, seeds and nuts by pressing or chemical extraction. To produce yellow spreads, the manufacturer takes the oil and, by deliberately altering the chemical structure, makes the liquid into a solid and some of the polyunsaturates into saturates by a process called hydrogenation.

Nutrition experts and researchers are now concerned that the hydrogenation process may be hazardous to health and, in the longer term, responsible for some of the heart and circulatory diseases which polyunsaturates were originally supposed to reduce.[2]

Hydrogenated spreads may also depress the immune system[3] and polyunsaturates have been linked, in animal studies, to skin cancer.[4]

Back to Butter

On the Food Combining Diet, butter and olive oil are classed as fats (neutral) and, in sensible amounts, are compatible with starches or proteins. It is worth remembering, however, that an excess intake of fats mixed with protein foods will delay and disturb protein digestion.

Butter is a high-fat food and so should be used sensibly in moderation but, on its own, is not responsible for heart disease. It is minimally processed and additive-free apart from some brands which contain salt. Butter adds a wonderful flavour to recipes and to bread and crackers. How many people do you know who swoon over hot polyunsaturated toast?

Anyone who does not like or is unable to use butter for any

reason could try the special spreads made from *un*hydrogenated oils which are available from health food stores. (See the Further Information list at the back of the book).

Healthy Olive Oil

Extra virgin olive oil is a monounsaturated oil, stable at room temperature and when heated and therefore suitable for cooking. It is also a flavourful base for salad dressings. Monounsaturates are now known to be a very healthy addition to a wholefood diet.[5,6,7] Although expensive, you will find that you use far less than other oils — and the extra flavour and health benefits are worth it. Store olive oil carefully in a cool dark cupboard away from heat and light.

Cream (Neutral/Fat)

Double, single, whipping and clotted creams are allowed — in moderation, of course — with proteins, starches, vegetable and fruit dishes.

The Problems of Low Fat Diets and Importance of Essential Fats

In an effort to lose weight, many dieters have chosen the low fat path. Cutting out all kinds of fat may induce impressive weight loss and used in the short term, they can be extremely effective. However, over the past three or four years, I have seen a stream of new patients — usually female — who have been using low fat (or no fat) diets as a way of life for long periods of time, certainly many months and in some cases years, afraid that, if they reintroduced fat into their menus, the weight would come romping back.

Although fat has been painted as an unrepenting villain in almost every discussion concerning heart disease, it is meant to form a natural part of any diet. When fat is removed from food (usually in an effort to reduce cholesterol or weight), fatty vitamins and some very important vitamin-like substances called *essential fatty acids* are also lost.

One of the main essential fatty acids, known as *linoleic acid (or LA)*, is found in nut, seed and vegetable oils but before it can be used internally, LA must be changed to *GLA (gamma linolenic acid)* by the body. Unfortunately, even when these oil-rich foods are abundant in the diet, the steps in the LA to GLA conversion process can be blocked by a variety of factors including stress, illness — particularly viral infections, high cholesterol and a typical Western diet which contains too many saturated and hydrogenated fats. There may be also an inherited inability in some people to convert LA to GLA biochemically. [8,9]

Essential fatty acids or EFAs form part of every single cell in the body and are needed for myriad body processes. Total abstinence from fat can result in joint stiffness, exacerbation of arthritis, skin problems, vaginal dryness (a particular problem in the post-menopause years), nervous disorders, twitchy limbs and an increase in susceptibility to viral infections, to name but a few.

The Food Combining Diet pays particular attention to the right kind of fats and oils, recommending extra virgin olive oil and small amounts of butter whilst avoiding the use of processed polyunsaturates and other high fat foods.

Fruits and Fruit Juices
(Alkaline Forming)

—— ॐ ——

Fresh fruits and fresh fruit juices are sources of concentrated energy which help the body to flush out accumulated toxic overload and waste products. They are the cleansers of the human system and are especially nourishing to a sluggish overweight body which is trying to shed a few pounds.

Fruits are an essential part of the Food Combining Diet but to be digested properly and to work efficiently must be treated with respect. All fruits prefer to be eaten entirely separately — not mixed with other food types such as proteins or starches. Trouble is, old habits die hard. Eating fruit as a dessert is commonplace — but isn't necessarily a good thing.

An apple, if eaten alone, will pass through the stomach in a relatively short space of time (15 to 20 minutes) whereas a heavy protein meal could remain there for 4 to 5 hours. If the apple is eaten on an empty stomach, it has free access to the small intestine, the next staging post in the digestive tract after the stomach. But if you eat that apple after a meal of, say, meat or eggs, one of two things will happen. Either the fruit will hasten the passage of the protein, which is then chased out of the stomach too quickly, or the protein will cause the fruit to stay too long in the stomach. Result? Fermented apple or incompletely-digested protein. Both cause havoc. One of the single most common causes of heartburn, indigestion and abdominal discomfort is taking fruit with or immediately after a main course.

Best Eaten Separately

The original Hay rules allowed for acid fruits to be combined with proteins and for very sweet ripe fruits to be mixed with starch but the combinations are very specific and can be confusing, especially considering that fruits, starches and proteins all require varying lengths of time to be digested.

The Food Combining Diet follows a very simple fruit rule. Eat fruits either completely on their own on an empty stomach or as a between meal snack, not with other foods or mixed with main meals.

As long as there are no starches or proteins included, most fruits will combine with each other because they are all alkaline-forming. In the Menus you will see that fresh fruit salads and dried fruit compotes only follow alkaline-forming salads which contain no protein and no starch. In any event, it is wise to take the extra precaution of leaving one hour between finishing your main course and beginning the fruit course.

Occasionally, treat yourself to an energy-packed breakfast of fresh fruit puréed with live yoghurt.

If you find the 'no fruit with meals' rule too difficult to follow, another way of separating fruit is the stacking method. Instead of the incompatible fruit being eaten straight after a meal, do it the other way around. Eat the fruit as a starter so that it arrives in the stomach first and can escape more easily and quickly to the small intestine before the arrival of other foods. It also helps to leave 15 to 30 minutes between starter and main courses if possible. Leaving space is a useful tip for hypoglycaemics too; it helps to even out erratic blood glucose.

Stewed fruit

Can cause severe digestive disturbance and so should be avoided if at all possible. Although Dr Hay included some cooked fruits in his recipes, his general view was that 'cooked fruits of any kind are dead foods'. 'Not that they do us harm in this form', he told us, but they do not contain the same levels of goodness as do raw fruits. Heat changes the chemistry. Cooking fruit makes it more acidic, important enzymes and vitamins are destroyed and the great value of the raw fruit is lost. [1]

All *raw fruit* is alkaline-forming once it has been absorbed and metabolized and this alkaline state acts to neutralize undesirable acids in the system. [2] If you particularly enjoy cooked fruit, it is best to limit intake to the occasional baked apple only.

Prunes and rhubarb are not included in the Food Combining Diet since they are both high in a substance known as oxalic acid. Oxalates are not only hard on the digestion but also bind to important nutritional minerals so that those minerals are lost from the body.

Dried Fruit

The way in which Dr Hay categorized *dried* fruit was to assess it according to its origin. For example, dried apple rings are prepared from fresh apples which are acid fruits so that both are happier to be associated with protein foods. Bananas — fresh or dried — are a sweet starchy fruit and will therefore mix with other starches. But don't let this confuse you.

Since the Food Combining Diet does not mix fruit with other foods anyway, such complications of having to work out which fruits are acid and which are sweet will not be necessary. I mention Dr Hay's classification here simply as a guide in case you decide to read about food combining in more detail from other books. It is, however, helpful to remember that, if you have recently eaten a starch meal, sweet dried fruits will be more compatible as the next course. If you have eaten a protein main course, then a fresh fruit salad of acid fruits would be more appropriate.

Since all fruits, dried or fresh, are alkaline-forming, they will mix well with each other as long as there is no starch or protein present. Check the fruit lists on pages 169–70.

Always check the labels on any dried fruit you buy. Most are sprayed with glazing agents and sulphur dioxide preservative which are best avoided. Glazing agents are mineral oils (mineral hydrocarbons) added to prevent vine fruits sticking together when packed and to give them an 'attractive sheen'.

These additives have had little toxicity testing but can accumulate in liver, spleen, lymph and fat tissue. Some health food stores and delicatessens supply unsprayed, additive-free dried fruits. Shelf life is shorter so buy in small quantities, store in a cool dry place and use up within a couple of months.

Fruit juices

Should be always diluted with one third filtered water and consumed on an empty stomach. In some countries, many types of commercial fruit juices contain additives and extra sugar which do not (as yet) have to be declared on the manufacturer's label. My recommendation to my own patients is to avoid packaged orange juice — however real or pure it proclaims to be!

Either squeeze your own or choose non–carbonated additive-free *apple or grape juice*.

Although some advocates of the Hay Way do not recommend *cranberry juice* because of its acidity, recent scientific research has proven the value of this old wives' remedy as an excellent preventative treatment for cystitis. To be of value, it must be fresh and unsweetened.

Juicing at home

If you have your own juicer machine, then you will know that juicing fresh fruit at home beats all ready-prepared juices into a cocked hat. For more information on juicing, have a look at the recommended reading list at the back of this book.

Pulses — A Special Case

⟡

Beans, Lentils, Chick Peas, Peas, Peanuts

(Pulses, also called legumes, are the edible seeds of the *Leguminosae* family of plants.)

Pulses have been the cause of some Food Combining confusion, having high concentrations of both starch and protein. Dr Hay classified them as starch but did not recommend them. Their acid-forming nature and notorious reputation for causing digestive havoc led him to the conclusion that they were best avoided. Indeed, they do not combine well with either starches or proteins and are well known for their gas-propelling properties. This is due to two particular carbohydrate (starch) molecules called raffinose and stachyose which are not dealt with properly in the upper part of the digestive tract, preferring to run amok, bloating abdomens and broadcasting sound effects, until they are broken down by the bacteria of the large bowel.

Problems with digestibility will be much more likely if the pulses are not properly prepared or mixed incorrectly with proteins or starches. If treated with respect, however, they have many beneficial attributes. To ban completely the use of pulses can be hard on vegetarians and vegans who do not, of course, eat flesh foods. Peas, beans and lentils provide valuable protein nourishment along with iron, calcium, zinc, magnesium and B vitamins.

Since it was discovered that the special kind of dietary fibre in pulses can help to regulate control of glucose in the blood, they have also been recommended for diabetics and hypoglycaemics. Another 'plus' for pulses is the fact that they can contribute to the production of butyric acid, a fatty acid which is formed during the breakdown of dietary fibre. Butyric acid is believed to be a factor in the prevention of colonic cancer.

Pulse Points

1. Do not mix pulses with proteins (meat, fish, eggs, milk etc.) or starches (potatoes, rice, pasta, bread or other grains).
2. Use the gas-free beans preparation method below — it helps to break down the troublesome raffinose and stachyose starches and destroys any anti-nutritional enzymes.
3. Eat pulses in small amounts only.
4. They mix well with all kinds of vegetables (except the few starchy ones) and salads.

Sprouted Pulses

When sprouted, the nutritional make-up of pulses changes completely. Easy and inexpensive to grow at home on a windowsill or in an airing cupboard, sprouts provide a very high level of nourishment and are naturally rich in amino acids, fatty acids, minerals and vitamins, particularly Vitamin C. For more information on sprouting, Leslie Kenton's best-seller *Raw Energy* is a must.

Gas-Free Beans!

1. Decide how many beans you need and check them over, removing any that are marked, damaged or discoloured.
2. Rinse them thoroughly through a sieve.
3. Soak them overnight in cool (filtered) water. Soya beans need a much longer soaking, usually 24 hours, and are best cooked in a pressure cooker. For soaking, you will need four measures of water to every one measure of beans.
4. After soaking, discard the water and rinse the beans several times in fresh water.
5. Place them in a large pan (not aluminium or copper) and cover them so that the water level is about 2 inches above the level of the beans. Add a tablespoon of cider vinegar.
6. Bring them to a fast boil. Any white scum which appears on the top is 'flatulence foam' so scoop it away and discard it.
7. Turn the heat down a little so that the beans are just bubbling but not boiling furiously.
8. Keep topping up the water level so that the beans remain well covered. Use boiling water from the kettle so that the pan does not go off the boil each time you top up.
9. Continue cooking in this way until the beans are easily broken when tested with a sharp knife. Cooking time will vary depending upon the type of bean so check with your own cookery reference or product pack.
10. Adding culinary herbs to the boiling liquid can help digestion too.
11. Always sit down to eat. Chew really thoroughly. Never eat beans late at night or when you are very tired.

Canned beans make a good emergency standby but don't forget to rinse them under running water before use.

Hummus

Hummus is a paste made with chick peas (garbanzos), garlic and sesame seeds and is categorized as a starch food. Although the Food Combining Diet does not recommend the mixing of pulses with other starches or with proteins, small amounts of hummus (say, one tablespoon) are acceptable as a topping for jacket potatoes.

Soya Beans And Soya Products Including Tofu, Tempeh, Miso, Soya Flour and Soya Milk

Soya products come under a separate heading from other beans and are listed as protein. Again, soya foods can be difficult for some people to digest and so should be taken in moderation only.

Menus

---------------- ❧ ----------------

When preparing vegetables and salads, always keep in mind
the 3 Ms:

Minimum cutting and chopping
Minimum water
Minimum cooking

Letter codes:
[A] = Alkaline-forming
[O] = Eat this entirely on its own
[P] = Protein
[S] = Starch
[V] = Suitable for vegetarians

Shopping

Check each day's menus in advance to see which ingredients you will need to put on your shopping list. Apart from fresh fruit and vegetables, some staples which are used regularly are:

- Black pepper
- Extra virgin olive oil
- Free-range eggs
- Garlic
- Sea salt
- Wholewheat pitta bread and yeast-free soda bread (both these breads keep well in the freezer)
- Oatbran or oatmeal and oatgerm
- Brown rice
- Soy sauce
- Plain live (bio) yoghurt — it is not necessary to choose the low-fat varieties
- Seeds:
    Pumpkin seeds
    Sunflower seeds
    Linseeds
- Dried fruit:
    Raisins
    Sultanas
    Dried figs
    Mixed dried fruit for fruit compote
- Nuts:
    Brazils
    Almonds — flaked and ground
    Pecans or walnuts
    Pine nuts

Week 1 Sunday

Starch Breakfast
FRUIT CIABATTA [S] [V]

or for a wheat-free breakfast
RICE CAKES WITH HONEY [S] [V] [WHEAT-FREE]

Ciabatta is a soft, open-textured bread made with olive oil. Available from most supermarket stores and good bread shops, it freezes well and thaws quickly so makes a good emergency standby. Most ready-made ciabatta breads come partly cooked and require further cooking of approximately 10 minutes in a hot oven. Best served hot with butter. The fruited ciabatta usually contains chopped walnuts as well as dried fruit.

Food Combining Guidelines: All types of bread and cereal are classed as starch so take care not to include any protein foods with this breakfast.

Pre-Lunch Aperitif
GLASS OF WHITE WINE OR FRUIT JUICE

Week 1

Protein Lunch
ROSEMARY'S ROAST LAMB WITH VEGETABLES [P]

I'm not going to insult anyone by telling them how to roast a joint or chop. Prepare lamb for the oven in your usual way and lay sprigs of rosemary over the joint. For a more pronounced rosemary flavour, make small cuts in the skin of the joint and push small sprigs of the herb into the meat.

When ready, serve with petits pois, green-headed broccoli (calabrese) or Brussels sprouts and parsnips. Eat as many vegetables as you like.

Food Combining Guidelines: Lamb is a protein so do not include any starch foods (i.e. potatoes or bread) at this meal. Although usually avoided by dieters because of its fat content, lamb is easier to digest than either pork or beef. Always choose lean cuts of organically-reared meat. This way you will cut down on the fat, avoid the drug and pesticide 'seasoning' so often associated with intensively-reared stock whilst still benefiting from a rich source of iron, zinc and B vitamins.

There is no gravy included with this meal. Most gravy recipes contain wheat flour — which is a starch and therefore incompatible with protein. Gravy can also be high in fat so try to avoid it if you can. Alternatively, look out for the excellent alternative gravy recipes in *Food Combining For Health* by Doris Grant and Jean Joice (Thorsons).

Alkaline-Forming Evening Meal
APPLE COLESLAW [A] [V]

Ingredients
1 chunk of a small white cabbage, shredded. How much you
    choose will depend upon your appetite.
1 medium-sized carrot, grated

1 grated apple
1 stick of celery, very finely diced
1 teaspoon chopped fresh chives if available
2 very finely chopped spring onions or green onions (called scallions in the United States)
2 grated Brazil nuts
1 teaspoon fresh lemon juice (for the apple)
1 tablespoon yoghurt dressing

The dressing
1 level tablespoon plain live yoghurt
1 spring onion (scallion) very finely chopped
1 clove of garlic — crushed
1 teaspoon fresh lemon juice
A little sea salt and freshly ground black pepper

- Blend the dressing by placing all the ingredients in a screw-top jar and shaking vigorously. Any leftover dressing will keep for a couple of days in the refrigerator.
- Prepare all the ingredients as above. Leave the apple until last and, once grated, cover it straight away with the lemon juice and mix thoroughly. Then stir all the ingredients together with the dressing and serve at once.

Tip: Coleslaw 'travels' well and makes a nutritious packed lunch. But, if you use it in this way, remember to take the whole apple with you and peel and slice it just before serving.

Watchword: Try to leave one hour between the main course and dessert.

Alkaline-Forming / Protein Dessert

FRESH PLAIN LIVE YOGHURT SWEETENED WITH A LITTLE HONEY
IF DESIRED [A] [P] [V]

Food Combining Guidelines: Yoghurt is a protein food but is also the only alkaline-forming dairy food which is readily available, all other kinds except raw unpasteurized milk being acid-forming. Don't mix yoghurt with starch.

Nutrition Plus: Fresh live additive-free yoghurt is super-nutritious and easy to digest, even for many of those who cannot tolerate cow's milk. Yoghurt provides valuable calcium, potassium, some zinc, B vitamins and Vitamin A plus those vitally important friendly flora which help to keep the gut healthy.

Week 1 Monday

Starch Breakfast
BANANA PORRIDGE [S] [V] [WHEAT FREE]

Use organic oatmeal or oatbran if possible. Using fine ground bran or meal and stirring the mixture throughout the short cooking time ensures a really smooth porridge which is easily digested.

Per serving: Take ½ cup of oatbran to 1½ cups of water. Place oatbran into pan and add the water, stirring until well mixed. Then place pan over heat and bring mixture to boil, stirring continuously. Turn down to simmer, still stirring all the time, for 2 minutes. Pour into a cereal bowl and decorate with sliced banana just before serving.

Food Combining Guidelines: This is a starch breakfast so don't be tempted to add any protein, ie milk.

Digestip: If you use rolled oat flakes instead of fine ground bran or meal, soak the oats overnight. They will be more easily digested.

Alkaline-Forming Midmorning Snack
KIWI FRUIT [A] [O] [V]

Alkaline-Forming Lunch
PINEAPPLE SALAD [A] [V]

Ingredients
3 slices of pineapple
1 large eating apple
1 stick of celery
1 tablespoon mixed pumpkin seeds and sunflower seeds

Cut the pineapple, apple and celery into cubes, mix together and sprinkle with the seeds. Add any coleslaw which is left over from yesterday.

Reminder: Don't forget to drink a glass of vegetable juice or water whilst preparing the evening meal.

Protein Evening Meal
BREAST OF CHICKEN SAUTÉED IN BUTTER AND SERVED WITH
CALABRESE (GREEN-HEADED BROCCOLI), CARROTS AND
MANGETOUT (SNOW PEAS) [P]

Sauté breast of free-range chicken gently in butter for 7–8 minutes each side (make sure it is cooked right through) and serve with as large a quantity of vegetables as you like.

Food Combining Guidelines: Chicken is protein so do not mix any starch foods with this evening meal!

Week 1 Tuesday

Starch Breakfast
HOME-MADE MUESLI [S] [V] [WHEAT FREE]

Ingredients
1 level tablespoon oatmeal or oatbran
1 level tablespoon of grated almonds (unblanched)
1 level tablespoon of grated Brazil nuts
1 level tablespoon of raisins
1 level tablespoon linseeds
1 level tablespoon pumpkin seeds
1 level tablespoon sunflower seeds
4 tablespoons of filtered water
1 tablespoon of lemon juice
2 tablespoons apple juice (not carbonated)
1 grated apple (grate immediately before serving)

Soak the oats in the filtered water and apple juice, cover, refrigerate and leave overnight. In the morning, grate the apple and mix it with the lemon juice. Add the soaked oats, seeds, nuts, dried fruit and apple juice. Serve with a little diluted cream.

Food Combining Guidelines: This delicious mixture is moist enough to eat without adding extra liquid. The addition of large amounts of milk to cereals is not recommended since milk is a protein and most cereals are starch-based, thereby making them incompatible. However, if at first you find it difficult to adjust, then add a little diluted organic raw milk or a small amount of diluted cream.

Alkaline-Forming Midmorning Snack
SMALL BUNCH OF GRAPES [A] [O] [V]

Alkaline-Forming Lunch
CRUDITÉS WITH AVOCADO DIP [A] [V]

Ingredients
Eat as many of these as you like depending upon how hungry
you are.

Slices of red, green and yellow peppers (capsicums)
Sticks of carrot, celery and cucumber
Cauliflower florets
Cherry tomatoes
Green onions (young spring onions; called scallions in the US)

Dip
½ avocado
Squeeze of fresh lemon juice
1 teaspoon extra virgin olive oil

Seasoning: a twist of freshly ground black pepper and sea salt
    Skin the avocado, remove the stone and mash the pulp with
the lemon juice, oil and seasoning.

Reminder: Are you drinking that glass of water or vegetable juice
whilst preparing the evening meal?

Protein Evening Meal
GRILLED LEMON SOLE WITH GREEN SALAD [P]

Before grilling, wash the fish and dry it on kitchen paper. To
enhance the flavour, moisten both sides with a little butter and
rub gently with a few sprigs of thyme.

To make the green salad:
Choose as wide a variety as possible of different green leaves,

depending upon the season. Here are some suggestions:

Beet greens; broadleaf Batavian endive; curly endive; Chinese leaves; dandelion leaves; radish leaves; rocket; spinach; cress and watercress; any kind of lettuce (butterhead; cos; crisphead or iceberg; lambs; lollo rosso; oak leaf; tango; curly leaf or Webbs).

When they are available, add fresh culinary herbs such as chervil; coriander; dill; fennel; marjoram; mint; oregano; parsley; sage or thyme.

Shred all the leaves into small pieces and dress with yoghurt dressing or olive oil dressing.

Food Combining Guidelines: The fish is protein so don't add any starch foods!

Week 1 Wednesday

Alkaline-Forming Breakfast
½ MELON [A] [O] [V]
(Use the other half tomorrow)

Food Combining Guidelines: Melon is best eaten completely on its own so don't mix it with any other food!

Alkaline-Forming Midmorning Snack
1 BANANA [A] [O] [V]
Banana is an alkaline-forming starchy fruit.

Starch Lunch
LEEK AND POTATO SOUP SERVED WITH RYE CRACKERS [S] [V]
[WHEAT FREE]

Ingredients
3 large potatoes (if organic, leave the skins on)
3 medium sized leeks
1 onion
1 level tablespoon oat bran
2 teaspoons extra virgin olive oil
Dried or fresh bouquet garni
1 teaspoon of fresh single cream to garnish
3-4 sprigs watercress or 3-4 fresh spinach leaves if available
Seasoning: freshly ground black pepper and sea salt to taste

- Finely chop the onion and fry it gently in the olive oil for 5 minutes.
- Cut the potato and leeks into small chunks and add them, with the oatbran and the bouquet garni to the pan.
- Cover with filtered water.

- Bring to the boil and then simmer until the potato is just cooked through but not soggy.
- Allow to cool sufficiently to liquidize safely.
- Prior to liquidizing, remove the herbs and add the watercress or spinach and seasoning.
- Dribble a teaspoon of fresh single cream over the soup before serving.

This recipe makes two very good-sized portions. Use half today and keep the remainder, covered and refrigerated, for tomorrow's lunch. If the weather does not call for hot soup, by all means change this meal to a preferred choice; perhaps a rice salad or rice crackers spread with avocado.

Food Combining Guidelines: The potato and oat bran in the soup, rye crackers (and rice) are all starch foods so no protein should be mixed with this lunch!

Reminder: Whilst preparing the evening meal, drink a glass of vegetable juice or water.

Protein Evening Meal
MUSHROOM AND ONION OMELETTE WITH GREEN SALAD [P] [V]

Ingredients
2 large flat mushrooms
1 small onion
2 large free-range eggs
1 tablespoon milk (raw sheep's or goat's if possible)
2 teaspoons extra virgin olive oil
1 level teaspoon butter
1 teaspoon of freshly chopped chives if available
Ground black pepper and sea salt seasoning

- Finely chop the onion.
- Discarding the stalks, cut the mushrooms into strips.
- Fry the onion and mushroom gently in the melted oil and butter until the onion is tender.
- Remove from the pan.
- Beat the eggs and milk with the chives and the seasoning and pour into the same pan which you used to cook the onions and mushrooms. Just before the omelette has set, tip the onions and mushrooms over the egg mixture.
- Fold omelette in half and serve with salad.

To make the green salad:
As before, choose as wide a variety as possible of different green leaves, depending upon the season. Here are my suggestions:
Beet greens; broadleaf Batavian endive; curly endive; Chinese leaves; dandelion leaves; radish leaves; rocket; spinach; cress and watercress; any kind of lettuce (butterhead; cos; crisphead or iceberg; lambs; lollo rosso; oak leaf; tango; curly leaf or Webbs).
When they are available, add fresh culinary herbs such as

chervil; coriander; dill; fennel; marjoram; mint; oregano; parsley; sage; thyme.

Shred all the leaves into small pieces and garnish with yoghurt dressing or olive oil dressing.

Food Combining Guidelines: This evening meal contains eggs which are a protein food so don't add any bread, potatoes, rice, pasta or other starches.

Week 1

Week 1 Thursday

Alkaline-Forming Breakfast
½ MELON [A] [O] [V]

Food Combining Guidelines: Don't forget, melon prefers to be eaten alone.

Alkaline-Forming Midmorning Snack
1 BANANA [A] [O] [V]

Starch Lunch
LEEK AND POTATO SOUP WITH RYE CRACKERS
(as yesterday) [S] [V] [Wheat free] or starch alternative of your choice

Watchword: Make sure that the soup is thoroughly reheated.

Reminder: Have a drink of juice or water while you prepare the snow pea salad.

Protein Evening Meal
HOT SNOW PEA SALAD [P]

Ingredients
3 oz/75g/⅓ US cup trimmed snow peas (mangetout)
One quarter of any small crisp lettuce
3 oz/75g/⅓ US cup freshest bean sprouts
1 firm, ripe tomato, skinned (please see p.154)
3 oz/75g/⅓ US cup peeled prawns
1 teaspoon soy sauce
1 teaspoon freshly chopped dill
1 teaspoon freshly chopped chives
3 button mushrooms
2 teaspoons extra virgin olive oil

Arrange the lettuce leaves on a large plate or serving dish. Melt the olive oil in a wok or skillet. Add all ingredients (except the lettuce) and stir-fry for 2-3 minutes, shaking the pan continuously. Tip ingredients onto the lettuce bed and serve immediately.

Food Combining Guidelines: This supper contains protein (peeled prawns) so don't add any starch foods to the recipe!

Week 1 Friday

Protein Breakfast
2 FREE-RANGE BOILED EGGS [P] [V]

Food Combining Guidelines: Eggs make a protein breakfast so no toast or rolls!

Alkaline-Forming Midmorning Snack
2 TABLESPOONS OF MIXED SUNFLOWER AND PUMPKIN
SEEDS [A] [V]

Starch Lunch
WHOLEWHEAT PITTA BREAD FILLED WITH LETTUCE,
WATERCRESS AND SLICES OF SKINNED TOMATO AND
CUCUMBER [S] [V]

Digestip: Throughout these menus you will see that any tomatoes used are always fresh, uncooked and skinned. I first began skinning tomatoes when my husband was convalescing; he was enjoying salads but finding tomato skin difficult to digest. In our view, skinning them not only improves digestibility but also enhances the flavour. It's quick and easy to do and no significant fibre or nourishment is lost. Turn to page 154 for the method.

Alkaline-Forming Evening Meal
RAW VEGETABLE FEAST [A] [V]

Reminder: Don't forget that all-important glass of vegetable juice or water to enjoy while preparing this meal.

Salad Ingredients

Carrot; celery; cucumber; tomatoes (skinned); radishes; wedges of Chinese leaves or iceberg lettuce; slices of red, green and yellow peppers.

Cut the celery, cucumber and carrot into slices or chunks and mix with the radishes, sliced peppers, sliced tomatoes and lettuce. Eat as much as you like.

If possible, leave one hour before enjoying:

Alkaline-Forming Dessert
FRESH FRUIT SALAD [A] [V]

Here are some fresh fruity suggestions for you to choose from:

apples; apricots; blackberries; blackcurrants; blueberries; boysenberries; carambola; cherries; clementines; grapefruit; grapes; huckleberries; kiwi fruits; loganberries; lillypilly fruits; lychees; mangoes; mulberries; nectarines; papaya; passionfruit; peaches; pears; pepino; persimmon; pineapple; pomegranate; raspberries; satsumas or strawberries.

Food Combining Guidelines: No protein or starch to be included at this purely alkaline-forming meal.

Week 1 Saturday

Alkaline-Forming Breakfast
ANY ONE KIND OF FRUIT IN ANY QUANTITY

Choose from: apples; apricots; blackberries; blackcurrants; blueberries; boysenberries; carambola; cherries; clementines; grapefruit; grapes; huckleberries; kiwi fruits; loganberries; lillypilly fruits; lychees; mangoes; melon — honeydew melon, cantaloupe melon or watermelon; mulberries; nectarines; papaya; passionfruit; peaches; pears; pepino; persimmon; pineapple; pomegranate; raspberries; satsumas or strawberries.

Try to stick to one kind of fruit at a time, say 2 apples or 2 kiwis for example (mixed fruit salads are really only for sweet treats). Have a different fruit for your midmorning break and different again for lunch. [A] [V]

Watchword: Don't forget to drink plenty of water throughout the day between meals.

Alkaline-Forming Lunch
CHOOSE A FRUIT-ONLY LUNCH FROM THE LIST ABOVE. YOU CAN ALSO DIP INTO THE SAME LIST IF YOU ARE PECKISH BETWEEN MEALS TODAY.

Starch Evening Meal
SAUTÉED POTATOES WITH GREEN SALAD [A] [S] [V]

Ingredients
1 large organic potato (two if you are hungry)
1 tablespoon extra virgin olive oil
Sea salt

Scrub the potato well and cut into 7 or 8 thick slices. Cook in the hot olive oil for 5 or 6 minutes each side or until golden brown. Sprinkle with sea salt and serve with the green salad.

To make the green salad:
   From this list, try to choose as wide a variety as possible of different green leaves, depending upon the season
   Beet greens; broadleaf Batavian endive; curly endive; Chinese leaves; dandelion leaves; radish leaves; rocket; spinach; cress and watercress; any kind of lettuce: (butterhead; cos; crisphead or iceberg; lambs; lollo rosso; oak leaf; tango; curly leaf or Webbs).
   When they are available, add fresh culinary herbs such as chervil; coriander; dill; fennel; marjoram; mint; oregano; parsley; sage; thyme.
   Shred all the leaves into small pieces. Add French dressing if liked.
   If possible, wait one hour after the main course before eating dessert.

Starch Dessert
CHOCOLATE POLENTA [S]

A quick-to-make custard dessert
You will need:

3 level tablespoons of polenta mix (corn meal)
1 teaspoon vanilla essence
1 tablespoon honey or real maple syrup
1 tablespoon grated carob
1 tablespoon flaked almonds
1 cup filtered water
¼ cup milk
pinch of mixed spice

- Stir the polenta, honey or syrup, mixed spice and vanilla essence together in a large heatproof bowl.
- Then mix the milk and water in a pan, heat quickly and remove from heat just before it boils.
- Pour the hot liquid slowly over the polenta, stirring until smooth.
- Return the mixture to the pan and continue stirring until you have a custard texture.
- Serve hot or cold, sprinkled with grated carob and flaked almonds.

Week 2 Sunday

Alkaline-Forming Breakfast
MANGO OR PAPAYA SLICES [A] [V]

Peel and slice a fresh mango or fresh papaya.

Food Combining Guidelines: This is a fruit-only alkaline breakfast so should have neither starch nor protein mixed with it.

Protein Lunch
TURKEY BREAST WITH GARLIC AND PARSLEY BUTTER SERVED WITH SALAD [P]

Ingredients
1 plump piece of free-range turkey breast
1 clove fresh garlic
1 teaspoon butter
½ teaspoon finely chopped fresh (or crushed dried) parsley
1 teaspoon extra virgin olive oil
4 crisp lettuce leaves (Webbs or iceberg) cut into strips
1 sliced skinned tomato (see page 154)
6 slices of cucumber (discard skin)
2 young spinach leaves or dandelion leaves finely shredded

To prepare the poultry: Crush the garlic clove and mix with the parsley and the butter. Slice the breast meat lengthways and spread the garlic mixture into the opening. Melt the olive oil in a fry pan. Add the turkey and simmer gently for 7–8 minutes (making sure it is cooked completely through). Shake the pan to prevent sticking and turn the meat a couple of times during cooking.

To prepare the salad: Arrange the green leaves in a serving dish and cover with the slices of tomato and cucumber.

Food Combining Guidelines: This is a protein meal (because of its poultry content) and therefore contains no starch.

Starch Evening Meal
BRAZIL BASMATI [S] [V]

Ingredients
1 cup of cooked brown basmati rice
1 tablespoon chopped Brazil nuts
1 onion
1 heaped tablespoon seedless raisins
1 level tablespoon sunflower seeds
1 teaspoon extra virgin olive oil

Chop the onion very finely and cook in the olive oil. When tender, add the cooked rice, nuts, raisins and seeds and stir until heated thoroughly. Serve with a green salad.

Food Combining Guidelines: It is the rice content which makes this a starch meal.

Watchword: Wait an hour before eating dessert.

Starch/Alkaline-Forming Dessert
BANANA AND ALMOND SMOOTHIE [A] [S] [V]

Ingredients
1 ripe banana
1 heaped tablespoon ground almonds
1 tablespoon fresh single cream
2 drops vanilla essence
1 teaspoon honey
1 tablespoon filtered water

Liquidize all the ingredients together in a blender.

Week 2

Week 2 Monday

Starch Breakfast
HONEY PORRIDGE [S] [V] [WHEAT FREE]

Use organic oatmeal or oatbran if possible. Using fine ground bran or meal and stirring the mixture throughout the short cooking time ensures a really smooth porridge which is easily digested.

Per serving: Take ½ cup of oatbran to 1½ cups of water. Place oatbran into pan and add the water, stirring until well mixed. Then place pan over heat and bring mixture to boil, stirring continuously. Turn down to simmer, still stirring all the time, for 2 minutes. Add one teaspoon of best quality dark honey just before serving.

Digestip: If you use rolled oat flakes, soaking them overnight will help to make them more digestible.

Food Combining Guidelines: Don't mix any protein with this starch breakfast!

Alkaline-Forming Midmorning Snack
APPLE OR PEAR [A] [O] [V]

Protein Lunch
SOFT CHEESE AND FRUIT SALAD [P] [V]

Ingredients
¼ avocado
1 stick of celery
1 crisp eating apple
1 ripe eating pear
1 tablespoon chopped pecan nuts
2 tablespoons of low fat soft cheese

Wash, peel and dice the pear and apple. Cut the celery into small pieces. Mix with all the other ingredients.

The rest of the avocado will be needed tomorrow so wrap the remainder and keep it in the refrigerator.

Food Combining Guidelines: The cheese makes this meal a protein one — so it contains no starch.

Reminder: Enjoy a glass of juice or water whilst preparing the stir-fry.

Alkaline-Forming Evening Meal
CRISPY VEGETABLE STIR-FRY [A] [V]

Slice the following ingredients into thin strips:

1 small onion
Red, green and yellow peppers
Shredded Chinese cabbage leaves
Thinly sliced cucumber
Carrot
Celery
Button mushrooms
Beansprouts or any other sprouted seeds
Cauliflower and/or broccoli, broken into small florets
Finely sliced fresh ginger
Extra virgin olive oil for stir-frying
A few drops of soy sauce

Fry the onion in 1 teaspoon of extra virgin olive oil. Add the ginger and the longer cooking vegetables (carrot, cauliflower, broccoli, celery, pepper) and stir-fry for 2 minutes. Then add the mushrooms, beansprouts, Chinese leaves, soy sauce and cucumber, stirring for a further 2 minutes. Season with black pepper and sea salt.

Food Combining Guidelines: This is an alkaline-forming meal containing no starch and no protein.

Week 2 Tuesday

Alkaline-Forming/Protein Breakfast
KIWI FRUIT FOLLOWED BY 1 SMALL TUB FRESH LIVE YOGHURT
[A] [P] [V]

Alkaline-Forming Midmorning Snack
ANY KIND OF FRESH FRUIT EXCEPT BANANA [A] [O] [V]

Protein Lunch
SLICED AVOCADO WITH 4 LARGE PRAWNS [P]

(This is the avocado left over from yesterday)
  Individual large prawns are sold by most fishmonger shops
and supermarkets.

Food Combining Guidelines: No starch at this meal; the prawns
are protein!

Starch Evening Meal
PINE NUT PASTA WITH WINTER OR SUMMER SALAD [S]

Ingredients
1 small onion
1 tablespoon extra virgin olive oil
1 tablespoon pine nuts
4 oz / 110g / ½ US cup of wholewheat spaghetti
Fresh marjoram, chopped, if available.

To make this supper wheat free and gluten free, choose rice spaghetti. (Details in information section at back of book.)

For any pasta use always the largest pan (no lid required) and plenty of water. Drop the pasta into the bubbling water and add a knob of butter or dribble of olive oil to help prevent it boiling over.

In a separate pan, fry the finely chopped onion in the olive oil. Once the pasta is cooked, drain the water away and tip the pasta into the onion pan with the pine nuts and chopped herbs, stirring it very gently two or three times before serving with the salad.

For Summer and Winter Salads, see page 156.

Food Combining Guidelines: Wholewheat pasta is a starch so no protein appears with this meal.

Week 2 Wednesday

Alkaline-Forming / Protein Breakfast
SLICED APPLE FOLLOWED BY FRESH LIVE YOGHURT [A] [P] [V]

Alkaline-Forming Midmorning Snack
1 BANANA [A] [O] [V]

Starch Lunch
TOMATO AND AVOCADO SODA BREAD [S] [V]

3 slices of wholewheat yeast-free soda bread spread with mashed avocado and slices of skinned tomato (see page 154).

Protein Evening Meal
GRILLED MACKEREL FILLET [OR WILD SALMON STEAK] WITH
SUMMER OR WINTER SALAD [P]

Summer salad p.156

Winter salad p.156

Food Combining Guidelines: The fish content makes this a protein meal so it has no starch included.

In advance: Prepare the dried fruit compote for tomorrow's breakfast.

Week 2 Thursday

Alkaline-Forming Breakfast
DRIED FRUIT COMPOTE [A] [V]

Choose any combination of these dried fruits: Apple rings; Yellow Apricots; Hunza Apricots; Banana; Currants; Dates; Figs; Pears; Seedless Raisins; Sultanas.

You will also need:

½ teaspoon cinnamon
2 cloves
1 tablespoon flaked almonds

Rinse the dried fruit thoroughly. Place in a pan (preferably stainless steel; not copper or aluminium) with enough filtered water to cover the fruit. Add cinnamon and cloves. Stir well, bring quickly to the boil and then remove from the heat. Cover the pan and leave to cool overnight. Serve with flaked almonds.

Food Combining Guidelines: Although some of these ingredients are from acid fruits and others from sweet (starchy) fruits, they are all alkaline-forming and therefore compatible with each other.

Alkaline-Forming Midmorning Snack
HANDFUL OF SUNFLOWER AND PUMPKIN SEEDS [A] [V]

Starch Lunch
PARSNIP AND NUTMEG SOUP [S] [V] SERVED WITH RYE CRACKERS [S] [V] OR YEAST-FREE SODA BREAD [S] [V]

Ingredients

1 small onion
6 young parsnips
2 medium sized potatoes (if they are organic, leave the skins on)
1 teaspoon ground nutmeg
1 tablespoon fresh single cream
1 tablespoon extra virgin olive oil
Seasoning: ground black pepper and sea salt

- Finely chop the onion and fry it gently in the olive oil for 5 minutes.
- Cut the potatoes and parsnips into small chunks and add them, with the nutmeg, to the pan.
- Cover with filtered water.
- Bring to the boil and then simmer until the parsnips are tender.
- Season.
- Retain all the liquid.
- Allow to cool sufficiently to liquidize safely.
- Stir in the cream before serving.

This recipe makes two very good-sized portions. Use half today and keep the remainder, covered and refrigerated, for tomorrow's lunch. In hot weather, this soup is just as delicious served chilled.

Food Combining Guidelines: The potato in the soup and the accompanying rye crackers or bread make this a starch lunch so no protein food is included.

Week 2

Protein Evening Meal
SARDINE AND TOMATO SALAD [P] [V]

Ingredients
1 small can (usual weight is around 100g to 120g) of sardines
   (in water or brine, not oil)
2 ripe, skinned, tomatoes
1 teaspoon finely chopped basil leaves
2 teaspoons extra virgin olive oil
1–2 teaspoons organic cider apple vinegar

Skin the tomatoes in the usual way (see p.154), laying the slices in a serving dish. Mix the olive oil, cider vinegar and basil thoroughly together and pour over the tomatoes. Serve with the sardines.

Food Combining Guidelines: The sardine content makes this evening meal a protein one.

Week 2 Friday

Protein Breakfast
2 POACHED EGGS WITH GRILLED MUSHROOMS [P]

Alkaline-Forming Midmorning Snack
4 DRIED FIGS [A] [O] [V]

Starch Lunch
PARSNIP AND NUTMEG SOUP WITH RYE CRACKERS OR SODA
BREAD [S] [V] [WHEAT FREE]
(as yesterday)

Alkaline-Forming Evening Meal
RAW VEGETABLE FEAST [A] [V]

Reminder: Don't forget that all-important glass of vegetable juice or water to enjoy while preparing this meal.

Salad Ingredients
Carrot; celery; cucumber; tomatoes (skinned); radishes; wedges of Chinese leaves or iceberg lettuce; slices of red, green and yellow peppers.

Cut the celery, cucumber and carrot into slices or chunks and mix with the radishes, sliced peppers, sliced tomatoes and lettuce. Eat as much as you like.

Watchword: Try to leave one hour between the main course and the dessert.

Alkaline-Forming Dessert
FRESH FRUIT SALAD [A] [V]

Choose from: apples; apricots; blackberries; blackcurrants; blueberries; boysenberries; carambola; cherries; clementines; grapefruit; grapes; huckleberries; kiwi fruits; loganberries; lillypilly fruits; lychees; mangoes; mulberries; nectarines; papaya; passionfruit; peaches; pears; pepino; persimmon; pineapple; pomegranate; raspberries; satsumas or strawberries.

Food Combining Guidelines: No protein or starch to be included at this purely alkaline-forming meal.

Week 2 Saturday

Breakfast
ANY ONE KIND OF FRUIT IN ANY QUANTITY
Choose from list given for Friday dessert.

Remember to stick to one kind of fruit at a time, say 2 pears or a bowl of cherries or strawberries for example. Have a different fruit for your midmorning break and different again for lunch. [A] [O] [V]

Watchword: Don't forget to drink plenty of water throughout the day between meals.

Alkaline-Forming Lunch
CHOOSE A FRUIT-ONLY LUNCH FROM THE LIST ABOVE. YOU CAN ALSO DIP INTO THE SAME LIST IF YOU ARE PECKISH BETWEEN MEALS TODAY.

Starch Evening Meal
THE MARSDEN SALAD [S] [V]
This salad was devised especially for my patients as a wonderful detoxifier, cleansing of lymph and liver. It was one of these patients who named it the 'Marsden Salad'.

Salad Ingredients

Grated raw beetroot; celery; carrot; dandelion leaves; watercress; Spanish onion; sprouted fenugreek seeds; sprouted alfalfa seeds; 1 garlic clove (crushed); 1 teaspoon chopped chives.

You will also need:

1 cup of cooked brown rice
olive oil and lemon juice dressing
black pepper and sea salt to season

Simply tear all the leaves into small pieces, chop the carrot, celery, beetroot and onion and mix with the rice, seeds, chives, crushed garlic and dressing.

Food Combining Guidelines: The rice content makes the Marsden Salad a starch meal. Remove the rice and it will be an alkaline-forming meal.

Watchword: Try to leave one hour between main course and dessert.

Starch/Alkaline-Forming Dessert
BANANA AND RAISIN CREAM [A] [S] [V]

1 large ripe banana
1 tablespoon fresh single cream
1 heaped teaspoon seedless raisins
1 heaped teaspoon sunflower seeds
1 tablespoon filtered water

Simply mix all the ingredients together in a blender.

Week 3 Sunday

Alkaline–Forming Breakfast
LARGE BUNCH FRESH GRAPES [A] [V]

Protein Lunch
**ROASTED FREE-RANGE CHICKEN SERVED WITH BUTTERED
BROCCOLI AND CAULIFLOWER [P]**

This is simply roast chicken with steamed vegetables, garnished with a little butter. If you are preparing the meal for one, buy a large breast of free range chicken on the bone and there will be enough for today's meal and tomorrow's lunch.

Food Combining Guidelines: Chicken is protein so no potatoes or other starch with this meal.

Starch Evening Meal
PASTA WITH PESTO [S] [V]

Ingredients
4 oz/110g/½ US cup of wholemeal pasta of your choice — any shape. I prefer to use Fusilli Bucati, the twisted spiral shape, fresh if possible — but dried is perfectly acceptable.
4 tablespoons extra virgin olive oil
2 cloves crushed garlic
1 tablespoon fresh chopped basil leaves
1 tablespoon pine nuts

To make the pesto sauce:
   Place the pine nuts, basil leaves, garlic and 2 tablespoons of olive oil in a food processor and blend until well mixed. Leave the machine running and, very gradually, add the remaining oil. Pesto will keep fresh for about 10 days if refrigerated in a screw-top glass container.
   Cook the pasta in the usual way, remembering to use a large pan with plenty of water. Pasta spirals cook very quickly.
   Toss the cooked pasta and prepared pesto sauce in a hot wok or pan just before serving. Can be accompanied with any green salad items.

Food Combining Guidelines: Pasta is, of course, a starch so no cheese (which is protein) should be included in this dish. If you are still hungry after the pasta meal, enjoy a few dates or some oatcakes with honey. Both are suitable after a starch main course.

Week 3 Monday

Alkaline-Forming Breakfast
½ FRESH GRAPEFRUIT FOLLOWED BY GRILLED
MUSHROOMS [A] [V]

Take 4 large flat mushrooms and brush both sides with a little
melted butter. Grill for 2-3 minutes.

Protein Lunch
SLICED COLD CHICKEN [P] WITH SUMMER OR WINTER SALAD
(SEE PAGES 156)

Alkaline-Forming Evening Meal
MIXED VEGETABLE SAUTÉE [A] [V]

Ingredients
1 small head of calabrese
1 quarter of a small cauliflower
2 carrots
2 leeks
1 tablespoon pine nuts
1 teaspoon of butter
4 tablespoons water
A little chopped mint
A few drops of soy sauce

Cut the vegetables into small pieces. Toss them in the melted
butter, add the water and leave them to cook gently with the
pan lid on tight.

Keep an eye on them. Vegetables can go from a state of
delicious just-cooked-crispness to unappetisingly-soggy in an
instant. When ready, sprinkle with the pine nuts, mint and soy
sauce.

Week 3 Tuesday

Alkaline-Forming / Protein Breakfast
SLICED FRESH APPLE FOLLOWED BY 1 SMALL TUB FRESH LIVE
YOGHURT [A] [P] [V]

Starch Lunch
TWO WHOLEWHEAT PITTA BREADS FILLED WITH HUMMUS [S] [V]

Time saver: If time is short, use ready-prepared hummus, now
available from most grocery stores, supermarkets and health
food shops. My own particular favourite home-made hummus
is Jackie Le Tissier's recipe in *Food Combining For Vegetarians*.

Protein Evening Meal
GRILLED TROUT WITH ALMONDS SERVED WITH TOMATO AND
DILL SALAD [P]

You will need:

1 small trout — cleaned and with head removed
1 tablespoon blanched, halved almonds
2 ripe, skinned tomatoes
1 tablespoon extra virgin olive oil
1 teaspoon finely chopped dill
2 teaspoons organic cider apple vinegar

- Skin and slice the tomatoes, laying them in a serving dish.
  Mix olive oil, vinegar and dill and pour over the tomatoes.
- Wipe the fish. Spread the inside with the butter and push
  in the almonds — they will stick to the butter.
- Grill the fish in the usual way and serve with the salad.

Food Combining Guidelines: This is a protein meal and so should
not include any starch.

Week 3 Wednesday

Alkaline-Forming / Protein Breakfast
PINEAPPLE LINSEED YOGHURT [A] [P] [V]

2 pineapple slices
1 tablespoon organic linseeds
1 small tub of live yoghurt

Blend the ingredients together until smooth.
Nutrition Plus: This mixture is easy on the digestion and wonderful for a sluggish bowel!

Starch Lunch
AVOCADO AND HUMMUS WITH CUCUMBER [S] [V]

You will need:
½ avocado
1 tablespoon hummus
6 slices skinned cucumber

Simply fill the avocado with the hummus and top with cucumber slices.
Food Combining Guidelines: Avocado and cucumber make this an alkaline-forming lunch but the addition of hummus changes the category to starch.

Alkaline-Forming Evening Meal
CRUNCHY NUT CALABRESE [A] [V]

You will need:

1 large head of calabrese
2 medium sized carrots
1 leek
2 courgettes (zucchini)
1 tablespoon sunflower seeds
2 tablespoons flaked almonds
1 teaspoon finely chopped mint
Knob of butter

This is a very nutritious supper, quick to prepare and ideal after a long day if you have no time to spend in the kitchen.

Slice the carrots and courgettes, chop the leeks into small chunks and break the calabrese into small florets. If the calabrese stalk is young and tender then slice this into thin strips. Discard if it seems tough. Sprinkle the vegetables with the mint and steam until al dente. Garnish with the butter, almonds, sunflower seeds and seasoning. Serve at once.

In advance: Prepare the Hunza apricots for tomorrow's breakfast.

Week 3 Thursday

Alkaline-Forming Breakfast
HUNZA APRICOTS [A] [V]

Take 8-12 Hunza apricots (depending upon your appetite). Rinse them thoroughly and place them in a stainless steel pan (not aluminium or copper). Add enough filtered water to the pan to cover the apricots. Bring quickly to the boil and remove from heat. Leave to cool overnight. No sweetening is required and the water will become delicious juice by morning.

Alkaline-Forming/Starch Lunch
'4P' SALAD WITH FRENCH DRESSING [A] [S] [V]

The four Ps stand for Pecan, Pine Nut, Pea and Potato.
  You will need:

2 tablespoons chopped pecan nuts
1 tablespoon pine nuts
2 tablespoons cooked petit pois (fresh or frozen but not dried
  or tinned)
8 oz/225g/1 US cup of cooked potato cut into small cubes.
  Choose organic potatoes if possible, so that the skins can be
  left on.

The dressing
1 tablespoon extra virgin olive oil
1 teaspoon finely chopped chives
1 very finely chopped spring onion (scallion)
1 teaspoon fresh lemon juice
A sprinkling of sea salt and freshly ground black pepper

Place all the dressing ingredients in a screw-top jar and shake vigorously.

Time saver: If you are in a hurry and cannot prepare this meal in advance, it is still as tasty if the peas and potatoes are just recently cooked and still hot.

Food Combining Guidelines: Potatoes make a starch meal but also a very healthy alkaline-forming one.

Protein Evening Meal
CHICKEN AND VEGETABLE KEBABS [P] OR EGG
RATATOUILLE [P] [V]

Ingredients for Kebabs
1 boned and skinned breast of free-range chicken
4 small button mushrooms (or larger ones halved)
1 courgette (zucchini)
½ red pepper
2 baby onions (or bulbs from spring onions), peeled
2 bay leaves
2 tablespoons extra virgin olive oil

- Cut the chicken, courgette and pepper into bite-sized chunks and thread them on to two lightly-oiled kebab skewers with the other vegetables and bay leaves.
- Brush lightly with the olive oil and season with a sprinkling or two of black pepper.
- Cook them under a hot grill, turning every two minutes, until the chicken is cooked through (about 10 to 12 minutes).

Ingredients for Ratatouille
2 tablespoons extra virgin olive oil
1 garlic clove, crushed
1 small onion, finely chopped
¼ each of red and green peppers, seeded and sliced
1 courgette (zucchini), topped, tailed and chopped
½ aubergine (eggplant), chopped
4 tablespoons dry white wine or water
2 teaspoons finely chopped fresh oregano
2 large tomatoes, skinned and chopped
2 free-range eggs

Heat the oil in a large saucepan and add the garlic and onion. Cook gently until the onion is translucent. Add the peppers, courgette, aubergine, liquid and herbs and stir to mix. Bring to the boil, then cover and simmer until the vegetabes are cooked through (about 15-20 minutes). Stir in the chopped tomato. Season to taste.

While the ratatouille is cooking, boil the eggs for about 10 minutes. Pour the prepared ratatouille into a serving dish and top with the halved eggs.

Food Combining Guidelines: Both chicken and eggs are protein — so no starch ingredients are included with the kebabs or the ratatouille.

Week 3

Week 3 Friday

Alkaline-Forming/Protein Breakfast
RASPBERRY AND LINSEED YOGHURT [A] [P] [V]

Ingredients
1 small tub of live yoghurt
1 tablespoon organic linseeds
4 oz/110g/½ US cup of raspberries either fresh or tinned in
    natural juice. Frozen raspberries are fine but you will need
    to remember to thaw them out overnight.

Blend all the ingredients together.

Alkaline-Forming Lunch
WALDORF SALAD WITH YOGHURT DRESSING [A] [V]

1 large apple, cored and diced
2 sticks celery cut into small pieces
A chunk of crispy lettuce, finely shredded
8 shelled walnut halves or pecan halves
½ avocado, sliced

The dressing
1 level tablespoon plain live yoghurt
1 spring onion (scallion) very finely chopped
1 clove of garlic, crushed
1 teaspoon fresh lemon juice
A little sea salt and freshly ground black pepper

Blend the dressing by placing all the ingredients in a screw-top
jar and shaking vigorously. Any leftover dressing will keep for
a couple of days in the refrigerator.

This is not a 'classic' Waldorf salad because of the avocado
content. Omit it if you like.

Alkaline-Forming Evening Meal
RAW VEGETABLE FEAST [A]

Reminder: Don't forget that all-important glass of vegetable juice to enjoy while preparing dinner.

Salad Ingredients
Carrot; celery; cucumber; tomatoes (skinned); radishes; wedges of Chinese leaves or iceberg lettuce; slices of red, green and yellow peppers; parsley sprigs.

Cut the celery, cucumber and carrot into slices or chunks and mix with the radishes, sliced peppers, sliced tomatoes and lettuce. Garnish with the parsley. Eat as much of this raw salad as you like.

Watchword: Leave an hour between main course and dessert if you possibly can.

Alkaline-Forming Dessert
FRESH FRUIT SALAD [A] [V]

Choose from: apples; apricots; blackberries; blackcurrants; blueberries; boysenberries; carambola; cherries; clementines; grapefruit; grapes; huckleberries; kiwi fruits; loganberries; lillypilly fruits; lychees; mangoes; mulberries; nectarines; papaya; passionfruit; peaches; pears; pepino; persimmon; pineapple; pomegranate; raspberries; satsumas or strawberries.

Food Combining Guidelines: No protein or starch to be included at this purely alkaline-forming meal.

Week 3 Saturday

Alkaline-Forming Breakfast
ANY ONE KIND OF FRUIT IN ANY QUANTITY

Choose from: apples; apricots; blackberries; blackcurrants; blueberries; boysenberries; carambola; cherries; clementines; grapefruit; grapes; huckleberries; kiwi fruits; loganberries; lillypilly fruits; lychees; mangoes; melon — honeydew melon, cantaloupe melon or watermelon; mulberries; nectarines; papaya; passionfruit; peaches; pears; pepino; persimmon; pineapple; pomegranate; raspberries; satsumas or strawberries.

Remember to choose only one kind of fruit. How about half a melon, a large bunch of grapes or a couple of peaches? Have a different fruit for your midmorning break and different again for lunch. [A] [V]

Watchword: Don't forget to drink plenty of water throughout the day between meals.

Alkaline-Forming Lunch
CHOOSE A FRUIT-ONLY LUNCH FROM THE LIST ABOVE. YOU CAN ALSO DIP INTO THE SAME LIST IF YOU ARE PECKISH BETWEEN MEALS TODAY.

Starch Evening Meal
TUSCAN SALAD WITH FRENCH DRESSING [S] [V]

Ingredients
1 cup of cooked brown rice
Slices of red, green and yellow peppers (capsicums)
2 green onions (young spring onions or scallions) finely chopped
2 oz/50g/¼ US cup of cooked broad beans
2 tablespoons of cucumber cut into small cubes
6 stuffed green olives

Mix all the ingredients together and serve with the dressing.
To make the dressing:

1 tablespoon extra virgin olive oil
1 teaspoon finely chopped chives
1 very finely chopped spring onion (scallion)
1 teaspoon fresh lemon juice
A sprinkling of sea salt and freshly ground black pepper

Place all the ingredients in a screw-top jar and shake vigorously.

Alkaline-Forming/Starch Dessert
BANANA AND ALMOND CREAM [A] [S] [V]

A quick and easy dessert.

You will need:
1 large ripe banana, 2 tablespoons flaked almonds, 1 tablespoon filtered water, 1 tablespoon fresh single cream, 3 drops vanilla essence.

Blend all the ingredients together and serve at once.

Week 4 Sunday

Starch Breakfast

4 DRIED FIGS [A] [V] FOLLOWED BY 4 RYE CRACKERS WITH HONEY
[S] [V]

Protein Lunch

POACHED FISH WITH MUSHROOMS [P] SERVED WITH SUMMER OR
WINTER SALAD [A]

Choose any kind of white fish and purchase enough for two
meals. Cook both portions and reserve one of them for
tomorrow's fish salad.

Apart from the fish, for today's lunch you will also need:

4 oz/110g/½ US cup of mushrooms
1 teaspoon butter
2 sprigs of thyme
2 tablespoons white wine
Filtered water

- Place the fish in a large pan and put in enough water just
  to cover it. Add the white wine and the thyme. Poach the
  fish gently until tender — probably only 2 to 3 minutes —
  and then remove from the heat.
- Remove one portion, allow it to cool and place it (covered)
  in the refrigerator ready for tomorrow.

- Chop the mushrooms very finely, fry them in the butter and use them to garnish the cooked fish.
- Serve with Summer or Winter Salad (see page 156).

Food Combining Guidelines: The fish makes this into a protein meal which could be served with green vegetables instead of salad but no potatoes, rice or pasta because these are classed under starch.

Leave one hour between main course and dessert.

Alkaline-Forming Dessert
BLACKBERRY AND APPLE 'CRUMBLE' [A] [V]

Ingredients
2 eating apples, grated
1 cup of fresh blackberries. If unavailable, use frozen blackberries or those which are tinned in natural juice.

To make the crumble, you will need:

1 teaspoon baking powder
1 heaped tablespoon sunflower seeds
1 heaped tablespoon pumpkin seeds
1 heaped tablespoon ground almonds
1 heaped tablespoon desiccated coconut
1 level tablespoon moist dark brown sugar
1 level tablespoon butter
1 tablespoon raisins

Place the apples and blackberries in a buttered pie dish. Using a food processor, mix the dry ingredients with the butter to the point where it resembles breadcrumbs. Mix with the raisins and tip the crumble over the apples and blackberries. Cook in a hot oven 400°F/200°C/Gas Mark 6 for 10-15 minutes or until topping is light golden brown. Serve with a little fresh cream.

Starch Evening Meal
NUTTY BROWN RICE [S] [V]

A quick, convenient and nourishing supper.

Ingredients

2 cups of cooked brown rice
1 leek cleaned, trimmed and finely chopped
1 tablespoon sunflower seeds
1 tablespoon pine nuts
2 tablespoons of canned sweetcorn or fresh baby sweetcorns halved
1 tablespoon extra virgin olive oil
6 or 8 mangetout
black pepper and sea salt to season

Fry the leek in the olive oil for 2 minutes. Then add the brown rice, mangetout and sweetcorn, stirring for a further 2 minutes. Sprinkle with the seeds, nuts and seasoning just before serving.

Tip: Many canned varieties of sweetcorn contain extra salt and sugar, so look out for 'no sugar, no salt added' brands and, before using, tip the can contents into a sieve and rinse thoroughly.

Week 4 Monday

Alkaline-Forming / Protein Breakfast
HONEY NUT YOGHURT [A] [P] [V]

Ingredients
1 small pot of plain live yoghurt
1 teaspoon of honey
1 teaspoon of oatgerm
1 teaspoon of crushed brazil nuts

Blend all the ingredients together.

Protein Lunch
FISH SALAD [P]

Take from the refrigerator the fish which you cooked yesterday, place it on a serving dish and coat it sparingly with yoghurt dressing. Sprinkle with black pepper and sea salt.

Serve with a mixed green salad. [A]

To make the green salad:

Depending upon season and availability, choose as many items as possible from this list:

Beet greens; broadleaf Batavian endive; curly endive; Chinese leaves; dandelion leaves; radish leaves; rocket; spinach; cress and watercress; any kind of lettuce (butterhead; cos; crisphead or iceberg; lambs; lollo rosso; oak leaf; tango; curly leaf or Webbs).

When they are available, add fresh culinary herbs such as chervil; coriander; dill; fennel; marjoram; mint; oregano; parsley; sage; thyme.

Shred all the leaves into small pieces and arrange them

on the fish platter. Add a little more dressing to the salad if desired.

Food Combining Guidelines: Fish is a protein food so this meal has no starchy ingredients.

Starch Evening Meal
BAKED JACKET POTATO TOPPED WITH HUMMUS [S] [V]

Accompanied by the Marsden salad, this is one of my favourite suppers.

Salad Ingredients
Grated raw beetroot; celery; carrot; dandelion leaves; watercress; Spanish onion; sprouted fenugreek seeds; sprouted alfalfa seeds. Dress with extra olive oil and cider vinegar.

Week 4 Tuesday

Starch Breakfast
FRUIT PORRIDGE [S] [V] [WHEAT FREE]

Use organic oatmeal or oatbran if possible. Using fine ground bran or meal and stirring the mixture throughout the short cooking time ensures a really smooth porridge which is easily digested.

Per serving: Take ½ cup of oatbran to 1½ cups of water.
You will also need:

1 tablespoon raisins
1 tablespoon sunflower seeds

Place oatbran into pan and add the water, stirring until well mixed. Then place pan over heat and bring mixture to boil, stirring continuously. Turn down to simmer, still stirring all the time, for 2 minutes. Add mixed dried fruit and sunflower seeds just before serving.

Digestip: If you use rolled oat flakes, soaking them overnight helps to make them more digestible.

Food Combining Guidelines: Don't mix any protein with this starch breakfast!

Starch Lunch
WHOLEWHEAT PITTA BREADS FILLED WITH ANY SALAD ITEMS OF
YOUR CHOICE [S] [V]

Food Combining Guidelines: Pitta bread makes this a starch meal.

Protein Evening Meal
VEGETABLE MEDLEY AU GRATIN [P] [V]

Choose vegetables from this list enough to provide one hearty serving: cauliflower, calabrese, carrot, leek, courgette, button mushrooms, swede and marrow.

You will also need:

1 tablespoon cashew nuts
2 oz/50g/¼ US cup of vegetarian hard cheese, grated

Cut all the vegetables into small pieces and steam until tender but not soggy. Serve with sprinkled nuts and cheese.

Food Combining Guidelines: The cheese makes this a protein meal.

Week 4 Wednesday

Starch Breakfast
HOME-MADE MUESLI [S] [V] [WHEAT FREE]

Ingredients

1 level tablespoon oatmeal or oatbran
1 level tablespoon of grated almonds (unblanched)
1 level tablespoon of grated brazil nuts
1 level tablespoon of raisins
1 level tablespoon linseeds
1 level tablespoon pumpkin seeds
1 level tablespoon sunflower seeds
4 tablespoons of filtered water
1 tablespoon of lemon juice or (still, not carbonated) apple
  juice
1 grated apple (grate immediately before serving)

Soak the oats in the filtered water, cover, refrigerate and leave overnight. In the morning mix the oats with the seeds, nuts, dried fruit and juice. Serve with the yoghurt.

Food Combining Guidelines: This delicious mixture is moist enough to eat without adding extra liquid. The addition of large amounts of milk to cereals is not recommended but if at first you find it difficult to adjust, then add a little diluted organic raw milk or a small amount of diluted cream.

Alkaline-Forming Lunch
NOURISHING VEGETABLE SOUP [A] [V]

Ingredients
2 medium-sized carrots
1 onion
1 small turnip
½ swede
1 leek
2 sticks celery
Fresh or dried bouquet garni
1 teaspoon soy sauce
1 teaspoon extra virgin olive oil

Chop the onion and cut all the other vegetables into small chunks. Place all the ingredients into a large pan with enough filtered water to cover them. Add the bouquet garni and simmer until the vegetables are tender. Remove the herbs and allow the mixture to cool sufficiently for safe blending with the soy sauce and olive oil.

You should have enough soup for two good-sized portions. Eat half today and refrigerate the remainder for tomorrow.

Food Combining Guidelines: This is a very nutritious, alkaline-forming snack. To make it a starch meal, you would add soda bread, pitta, toast or crackers.

Protein Evening Meal
SLICES OF VEGETARIAN CHEDDAR [P] [V] WITH WINTER OR
SUMMER SALAD [V]

See page 156 for Winter and Summer Salad recipes.

If vegetarian cheddar cheese is not available, choose any other kind of rennet-free vegetarian cheese.

Week 4 Thursday

Protein Breakfast
2 FREE-RANGE BOILED EGGS [P] [V]

Food Combining Guidelines: Don't forget that, because eggs are a protein food, you have to forego the bread or rolls at this meal.

Alkaline-Forming Lunch
NOURISHING VEGETABLE SOUP [A] [V]
(as yesterday)

Alkaline-Forming/Starch Evening Meal
BAKED JACKET POTATO WITH VEGETABLES [A] [S] [V]

Choose any vegetables from this selection to provide an ample serving: cauliflower, calabrese, carrot, leek, courgette, button mushrooms, swede and marrow. [A]

Cut the vegetables into small pieces and steam them. Serve with the jacket potato. A dressing of extra virgin olive oil and cider vinegar with chopped parsley adds extra flavour.

Food Combining Guidelines: This is a starch meal because of its potato content but is also alkaline-forming. Try to obtain organic potatoes so that you can eat the skin.

Week 4 Friday

Starch Breakfast

YEAST-FREE WHOLEMEAL SODA BREAD SPREAD WITH BUTTER
AND HONEY [S] [V]

Protein Lunch

GREEK SALAD [P] [V]

Ingredients
1 chunk of crisphead lettuce
4 green or spring onions (scallions)
1 ripe, skinned and sliced, tomato or 4 cherry tomatoes
6 slices of cucumber
6 black olives
2 oz/50g/¼ US cup of feta cheese cut into small cubes
6 small fresh mint leaves if available

For the dressing:

1 tablespoon olive oil
2 teaspoons fresh lemon juice

Shred the lettuce into fine strips and lay in a serving dish with
the mint leaves, tomato and cucumber slices, chopped onions
and the olives. Pour the dressing over and garnish with the
cheese.

Food Combining Guidelines: Greek salad is a protein meal
because of the cheese content.

Alkaline-Forming Evening Meal
RAW VEGETABLE FEAST [A] [V]

Salad Ingredients
Carrot; celery; cucumber; tomatoes (skinned); radishes; wedges
of Chinese leaves or iceberg lettuce; slices of red, green and
yellow peppers; parsley sprigs.

Cut the celery, cucumber and carrot into slices or chunks and
mix with the radishes, sliced peppers, sliced tomatoes and
lettuce. Garnish with the parsley. Eat as much of this raw salad
as you like.

Watchword: If possible, leave one hour between main course and
dessert.

Alkaline-Forming Dessert
FRESH FRUIT SALAD [A] [V]
Choose from: apples; apricots; blackberries; blackcurrants;
blueberries; boysenberries; carambola; cherries; clementines;
grapefruit; grapes; huckleberries; kiwi fruits; loganberries;
lillypilly fruits; lychees; mangoes; mulberries; nectarines;
papaya; passionfruit; peaches; pears; pepino; persimmon;
pineapple; pomegranate; raspberries; satsumas or strawberries.

Food Combining Guidelines: No protein or starch to be included
at this purely alkaline-forming meal.

Week 4 Saturday

Alkaline-Forming Breakfast
ANY ONE KIND OF FRUIT IN ANY QUANTITY.

Choose from: apples; apricots; blackberries; blackcurrants; blueberries; boysenberries; carambola; cherries; clementines; grapefruit; grapes; huckleberries; kiwi fruits; loganberries; lillypilly fruits; lychees; mangoes; melon — honeydew melon, cantaloupe melon or watermelon; mulberries; nectarines; papaya; passionfruit; peaches; pears; pepino; persimmon; pineapple; pomegranate; raspberries; satsumas or strawberries.

Choose one kind of fruit only. Have a different fruit for your midmorning break and different again for lunch. [A] [V]

Watchword: Don't forget to drink plenty of water throughout the day between meals.

Alkaline-Forming Lunch
CHOOSE A FRUIT-ONLY LUNCH FROM THE LIST ABOVE. YOU CAN ALSO DIP INTO THE SAME LIST IF YOU ARE PECKISH BETWEEN MEALS TODAY.

Protein Evening Meal
STIR-FRIED VEGETABLES AND WHITEBAIT [P]

Ingredients
1 tablespoon of extra virgin olive oil
A few drops of soy sauce
3 small sprigs of rosemary
¼ cup of each of the following:
  beansprouts
  shredded spinach
  chopped button mushrooms
  sliced red, green and yellow peppers (capsicums)
  thinly sliced courgette
  young spring onion (scallions) or Spanish onion
  pine nuts
  unblanched whole almonds
  12 whitebait

Using a wok or large skillet, stir-fry the whitebait in hot olive oil until they begin to turn crisp and brown (about 5 or 6 minutes). Keep shaking the pan to prevent sticking. Remove the fish from the pan and keep them hot. Stir-fry the remaining ingredients for 2–3 minutes. Just before serving, return the whitebait to the pan with the soy sauce. Mix and turn once or twice.

Watchword: Try to leave one hour between main course and dessert.

Week 4

Alkaline-Forming Dessert
RASPBERRY CREAM [A] [P]

Ingredients

1 cup of fresh, frozen (or tinned in juice) raspberries
  (put 4 raspberries to one side for decoration)
½ cup of fresh plain live yoghurt
1 tablespoon fresh single cream
1 teaspoon honey

Blend the ingredients to a smooth cream. Serve in a sundae
glass and decorate with the 4 whole raspberries.

Master Recipes

Tomatoes — The Marsden Way

Several of the recipes in this book contain tomatoes — fresh, raw and skinned *but never cooked*.

Those who find tomatoes difficult to digest have usually consumed them (complete with skins) in grills, sauces, purées or other cooked tomato dishes. If 'tomato indigestion' has compelled you to avoid this valuable fruit then try the Marsden way from now on.

Raw tomatoes are alkaline-forming and will mix happily with either starch (for example with wholemeal soda bread to make a delicious sandwich) or protein (perhaps with a cold chicken or egg salad). Once cooked, their acidity increases, making them completely incompatible with starch foods. In addition, their rich Vitamin C content is destroyed by prolonged heating.

If you think pasta without tomatoes is a crime, then try the fresh 'Love Apple' sauce on page 158 which needs no cooking.

ANCIENT HISTORY

The tomato's history began in South America where it was known as 'tomatl'. Its old European name 'love apple' descended from the Italian *pomo dei mori* and the French *pomme d'amour*. Botanically a berry fruit, the tomato is a member of the nightshade family and should be avoided by anyone who has an allergy to this particular family of foods.

STORAGE

Prolonged chilling interferes with texture and flavour so don't store ripening tomatoes in the refrigerator. Allow them to ripen naturally — away from direct daylight — at room temperature. Once fully ripened, they can be kept in the salad compartment of the refrigerator but should be used within 3 or 4 days.

SKINNING

The tomato's flavour — and its digestibility — is definitely improved by skinning. Here is my method:

Take a large heat-proof glass jug and put the tomatoes in it. Boil a kettle or pan of water and pour the just-boiled water over the tomatoes until they are completely submerged. Count 25 seconds — no more. Then pour the water away and remove the tomatoes from the jug. With a sharp knife, take a thin slice from the top of the tomato. As you cut, you will find that the remaining skin pulls away easily.

I have seen many descriptions of this simple process in cookery books which recommend leaving the tomatoes in the boiling water for 'a few minutes'. In my experience, this is far too long, begins to cook the tomato and risks the destruction of valuable vitamin C.

Tomato Salad [A] [V]

2 firm ripe tomatoes, skinned
1 teaspoon finely chopped basil
1 clove of fresh garlic, crushed
2 teaspoons of extra virgin olive oil
1 teaspoon of organic cider apple vinegar or
1 teaspoon fresh lemon juice
1 sprig of mint to garnish

Skin and slice the tomatoes. Place the basil, garlic, oil and vinegar or lemon juice in a screw-top jar and shake vigorously. Pour over the tomatoes and garnish with the mint.

Greek Salad [P] [V]

To make the Greek Salad, you will need:

1 chunk of crisphead lettuce
4 green or spring onions (scallions)
1 ripe, skinned and sliced, tomato or 4 cherry tomatoes
6 slices of cucumber
6 black olives
2 oz/50g/¼ US cup of feta cheese cut into small cubes
6 small fresh mint leaves if available

For the dressing
1 tablespoon olive oil
2 teaspoons fresh lemon juice

Shred the lettuce into fine strips and lay in a serving dish with the mint leaves, tomato and cucumber slices, chopped onions and the olives. Pour the dressing over and garnish with the cheese.

Food Combining Guidelines: Greek salad is a protein meal because of the cheese content.

Winter Salad [A] [V]

Ingredients
3 oz/75g/⅓ US cup finely grated white cabbage
1 medium sized carrot, grated
1 stick celery, very finely diced
1 eating apple, grated
1 teaspoon seedless raisins
1 tablespoon raw mild onion, finely chopped

Prepare all the ingredients and mix them together in a salad
bowl. If dressing is required, use olive oil, lemon juice and
seasoning to taste.

Summer Salad [A] [V]

Ingredients
4 sprigs of watercress
Chunk of crisphead lettuce
1 firm tomato, skinned and sliced
4-6 spinach leaves
6 slices of cucumber — discard the skin
¼ avocado, sliced
A few slices of red, green and/or yellow peppers
2 sprigs of fresh parsley

Slice the lettuce into fine strips and spread them over a serving
dish. Tear the watercress, parsley and spinach leaves into small
pieces and sprinkle them over the lettuce. Arrange the
remaining ingredients over this green base.

    If dressing is required, use olive oil, lemon juice and
seasoning to taste.

Green Salad [A] [V]

Ingredients

From this list, try to choose as wide a variety as possible of different green leaves, depending upon the season:

Beet greens; broadleaf Batavian endive; curly endive; Chinese leaves; dandelion leaves; radish leaves; rocket; spinach; cress and watercress; any kind of lettuce (butterhead; cos; crisphead or iceberg; lambs; lollo rosso; oak leaf; tango; curly leaf or Webbs).

When they are available, add fresh culinary herbs such as chervil; coriander; dill; fennel; marjoram; mint; oregano; parsley; sage; thyme.

Shred all the leaves into small pieces and add the appropriate dressing.

The Marsden Salad [A] [V]

Here is my lymph and liver detoxifier.

Salad Ingredients

Grated raw beetroot; celery; carrot; dandelion leaves; watercress; Spanish onion; sprouted fenugreek seeds; sprouted alfalfa seeds; 1 garlic clove (crushed); 1 teaspoon chopped chives.

To make this salad into a starch meal add:

1 cup of cooked brown rice
extra virgin olive oil and lemon juice

Simply tear all the leaves into small pieces and mix with the rice, seeds, chives, crushed garlic and dress with olive oil and lemon juice.

If you want to use this with a protein meal don't forget to omit the rice.

Love Apple Sauce

Wonderful with pasta!

Ingredients
1 small mild-flavoured onion
6 oz/175g/1 US cup of sweet, ripe tomatoes, skinned
2 teaspoons finely chopped fresh basil leaves
2 cloves fresh garlic, crushed
Freshly ground black pepper and sea salt to season
3 tablespoons extra virgin olive oil

Put the tomatoes, garlic, onion and seasoning into a blender and, with the motor running, add the olive oil at a slow trickle. Remove mixture from the blender and stir in the chopped basil.

If cold sauce doesn't appeal, simply place the mixture in a pan and heat it through as quickly as possible before pouring over the ready-to-serve pasta.

Food Lists

Foods to Combine at a Protein Meal

Nuts

+ Almonds
+ Brazil Nuts
- Candle Nuts
- Cashew Nuts
- Coconut
- Hazelnuts [Filberts]
- Macadamia Nuts
- Pecan Nuts
- Pine Nuts
- Pistachios
- Walnuts

Seeds

+ Caraway Seeds
+ Celery Seeds
+ Dill Seeds
+ Fennel Seeds
+ Fenugreek Seeds
+ Linseeds
+ Poppy Seeds
+ Pumpkin Seeds [Pepitas]
+ Sesame Seeds
+ Sunflower Seeds

Soya Protein — use sparingly

- Soya Beans
- Soya Flour
- Soya Lecithin
- Miso — caution, very high in salt
- Tempeh

– Tofu
– TVP – Textured Vegetable Protein

Soya–based products can be difficult for some people to digest. They should be treated as acid–forming protein, used in moderation only and not be mixed with either starches or sugars.

– Cheese

– Free Range Eggs

– Free Range Poultry

– Lean Lamb

– Lamb's Liver

– Rabbit

– Yogurt

Milk – see important notes on pages 59–61.

N Buttermilk
N Goat's Milk
N Sheep's Milk
N Semi–skimmed Cow's Milk – sparingly only
(Do not use UHT or homogenized cow's milk)
Condensed Milk – use very sparingly
Evaporated Milk – use very sparingly

All Kinds of Fish and Shellfish including

– Anchovies	– Eel
– Bass	– Haddock
– Cod	– Hake

- Coley
- Crab
- Dover Sole
- Halibut
- Herring
- Hoke
- Kipper
- Lemon Sole
- Mackerel
- Monkfish
- Mussel
- Oyster
- Prawns
- Pilchard
- Plaice
- Rainbow Trout
- Roe
- Salmon
- Salmon Trout
- Sardine
- Sea Cucumber
- Shrimp
- Tuna
- Whitebait
- Whiting
- Cod Liver Oil
- Halibut Liver Oil

Remember that all fish and shellfish is acid-forming.

Fats and Oils

N Butter
N Cream
N Non-hydrogenated [margarine-type] spreads
Hydrogenated vegetable fats should be avoided; see page 73.

Cold Pressed Oils

N Extra Virgin Olive Oil
N Hazelnut Oil
N Linseed Oil [Flaxseed]
N Safflower Oil
N Sunflower Oil
N Walnut Oil

Foods to Combine at a Starch Meal

Cereals and Grains (All acid-forming except millet)

- Barley
- Brown Basmati Rice
- Brown Rice
- Buckwheat
- Bulgur [Burghul]
- Corn [Maize]
- Couscous
- Cracked Wheat
- Macaroni
- Maize [Corn]
- Matzo Meal
+ Millet
- Oat Bran
- Oats

- Pasta
- Popcorn
- Potato Flour
- Quinoa
- Rice Bran
- Rice Flour
- Rye
- Rye Flour
- Tapioca
- Triticale
- Wholegrain Bread
- Wholemeal Flour
- Wild Rice

- Biscuits [cookies]
- Bread
- Cakes
- Crackers
- Pastry

Starchy Vegetables (All alkaline-forming)

+ Breadfruit
+ Potato
+ Pumpkin
+ Squash

+ Sweetcorn
+ Sweet Potato
+ Taro
+ Yams

Fats and Oils

N Butter
N Cream
N Non-hydrogenated [margarine-type] spreads
Hydrogenated vegetable fats should be avoided; see page 73.

Cold Pressed Oils

N Extra Virgin Olive Oil   N Safflower Oil
N Hazelnut Oil   N Sunflower Oil
N Linseed Oil [Flaxseed]   N Walnut Oil

Nuts	Seeds
+ Almonds	+ Caraway Seeds
+ Brazil Nuts	+ Celery Seeds
− Candle Nuts	+ Dill Seeds
− Cashew Nuts	+ Fennel Seeds
− Coconut	+ Fenugreek Seeds
− Hazelnuts [Filberts]	+ Linseeds
− Macadamia Nuts	+ Poppy Seeds
− Pecan Nuts	+ Pumpkin Seeds [Pepitas]
− Pine Nuts	+ Sesame Seeds
− Pistachios	+ Sunflower Seeds
− Walnuts	

Sweetenings — only in moderation

− Barbados Sugar   − Carob Spread
+ Blackstrap Molasses   − Crystallized Ginger
− Desiccated and Creamed Coconut
− Organic unblended honey
− Natural Maple Syrup [beware of imitations]
− Fructose [Fruit Sugar] — useful for baking (see note below)

Note: Fructose

Fructose has almost twice the sweetness of ordinary table sugar so only half the usual quantity is needed. Fructose doesn't require insulin for absorption and so puts less strain on the organs which control blood sugar — the pancreas, adrenals and liver. It is still a sugar, however, and should be used sparingly.

Neutral Foods

Vegetable List

I have included as comprehensive a list of vegetable foods as possible, with some of the popular Australian and American varieties for the benefit of readers in those countries. Different countries sometimes have different names for the same vegetable and so alternative names have been included where applicable.

These neutral foods will combine well with either starches or proteins — or as nutritious foods combined simply with each other. All are alkaline-forming except asparagus tips.

+ Alfalfa Sprouts
+ Artichokes
− Asparagus
+ Aubergine [Eggplant]
+ Avocado (strictly a fruit but listed here because it is so commonly used as a salad food)

+ Bamboo Shoots
+ Bean Sprouts
+ Beet Greens

+ Beetroot
+ Belgian Endive [Chicory]
+ Broadleaf Batavian Endive [Escarole]
+ Brussels Sprouts
+ Butterhead Lettuce

+ Calabrese [Green-Headed Broccoli]
+ Chinese Broccoli [Chinese Kale]
+ Purple Sprouting Broccoli

+ Cabbage: red, green or white
+ Capsicums: red, green or yellow [Peppers]
+ Carrots
+ Cassava
+ Cauliflower
+ Celeriac
+ Celery
+ Chayote [Choko, Vegetable Pear]
+ Chinese Cabbage [Chinese Leaves]
+ Cos lettuce
+ Courgette [Zucchini]
+ Cress
+ Cucumber

+ Dandelion Leaves

+ Eggplant [Aubergine]
+ Curly Endive
+ Escarole [Broadleaf Batavian Endive]

+ Garlic

+ Iceberg Lettuce

+ Kale [Collard]

+ Kohlrabi

+ Lamb's Lettuce
+ Leek
+ Lettuces [any kind]
+ Lollo Rosso

+ Mushrooms

+ Nettles

+ Oak Leaf Lettuce
+ Green Olives
+ Okra
+ Onion
+ Spanish Onion
+ Spring Onion
+ Scallions [young bulbless spring onions, also called green onions]

+ Parsnips
+ Peas
+ Sugar Peas
+ Mangetout [Snow Peas]

+ Radishes
+ Rocket
+ Romaine
+ Rutabaga [Swede]

+ Salsify
+ Silverbeet
+ Spinach
+ Sprouted Beans
+ Sprouted Seeds
+ Swede [Rutabaga]
+ Swiss Chard

+ Tango
+ Tomatoes (alkaline-forming when raw, acid-forming when cooked)
+ Turnips
+ Turnip Greens

+ Watercress
+ Webb's lettuce

+ Zucchini [Courgette]

Sea Vegetables [seaweed]

Seaweed is a general term for several kinds of sea vegetables. Some seaweeds have quite a strong taste so only a small amount is needed. Sold in its fresh state in some countries but more usually available dried from the health food store, it is used in soups and stews as an alternative flavouring to salt. Fat free and low in calories, seaweed is prized for its exceptional mineral content, being a rich source of calcium, iron and iodine with a valuable array of other trace minerals including zinc, manganese, chromium, selenium and cobalt. Unfortunately, it can be also rich in nitrates, strontium, cadmium, lead and mercury and so is, perhaps, less desirable than it once was.

+ Chinese Black Moss
+ Dulse
+ Hijiki
+ Kombu
+ Mekabu
+ Nori
+ Wakame

Herbs and Spices

Herbs and spices can be included with proteins or starches and with vegetables and salads. Use spices sparingly.

Herbs

+ Angelica
+ Anise [Aniseed]
+ Basil
+ Bay Leaf
+ Bergamot
+ Borage

+ Chervil
+ Chives
+ Coriander
+ Dill
+ Fennel
+ Fenugreek
+ Horseradish
+ Lemon Balm
+ Lemon Grass
+ Lemon Verbena
+ Lovage
+ Marjoram
+ Mint

+ Myrtle
+ Oregano
+ Parsley
+ Rosemary
+ Sage
+ Salad Burnet
+ Savory
+ Shiso
+ Tansy
+ Tarragon
+ Thyme
+ Yarrow

Spices

− Allspice
− Cayenne [Chilli]
− Cinnamon
− Cloves
− Cumin

− Ginger
− Liquorice
− Mustard
− Paprika
− Turmeric

Fats and Oils

N Butter
N Cream
N Non-hydrogenated [margarine−type] spreads
Hydrogenated vegetable fats should be avoided; see page 73.

Cold Pressed Oils

N Extra Virgin Olive Oil
N Hazelnut Oil
N Linseed Oil [Flaxseed]
N Safflower Oil
N Sunflower Oil
N Walnut Oil

Nuts

see notes on page 72.

+ Almonds
+ Brazil Nuts
− Bunya Bunya Pine Nuts
− Candle Nuts
− Cashew Nuts
− Coconut
− Hazelnuts [Filberts]
− Macadamia Nuts
− Pecan Nuts
− Pine Nuts
− Pistachios
− Red Bopple Nuts
− Tiger Nuts
− Walnuts
− Water Chestnuts

Seeds

+ Caraway Seeds
+ Celery Seeds
+ Dill Seeds
+ Fennel Seeds
+ Fenugreek Seeds
+ Linseeds
+ Poppy Seeds
+ Pumpkin Seeds [Pepitas]
+ Sesame Seeds
+ Sunflower Seeds

Fruit List

Fruits from this list will make for healthy alkaline-forming breakfasts, between-meal snacks, fruit-only lunches and (with the exception of melon) fruit salads. Remember to keep fruits away from proteins and starches.

I have included as comprehensive a list of fruits as possible. A few names may not be so familiar to UK readers but are included for the benefit of those in other countries. Where there is more than one popular name for a particular fruit, both have been listed.

+ Abiu
+ Apples (fresh and dried)
+ Apricots:
   Hunza Apricots (dried — available from health food stores)
   Yellow Apricots (fresh and dried)

+ Babaco
+ Banana (fresh and dried)
+ Blackberries
+ Blackcurrants
+ Blueberries
+ Boysenberries

+ Carambola [star fruit]
+ Cherries
+ Clementines
+ Cumquat [also spelled kumquat]
+ Currants

+ Dates

+ Figs (fresh and dried)
+ Granadillas
+ Grapefruit
+ Grapes
+ Guava

+ Huckleberries

+ Jackfruit

+ Kiwi Fruit

+ Lemons
+ Lillypilly Fruits
+ Limes
+ Loganberries
+ Lychees

+ Mandarins
+ Mangoes
+ Medlars
+ Melons (melon is best eaten on its own):

Cantaloupe Melon
Gallia Melon
Honeydew Melon
Horned Melon
Kiwano
Persian Melon
Rockmelon
Watermelon
+ Mulberries

+ Nectarines

+ Papaya [paw–paw]
+ Passionfruit
+ Peaches (fresh and dried)
+ Pears (fresh and dried)
+ Pepino
+ Persimmon [date plum]
(fresh and dried)

+ Pineapple
+ Pitahaya [cactus fruit]
+ Plantain
+ Pomegranate

+ Raisins
+ Raspberries
+ Redcurrants

+ Sapodilla
+ Satsumas
+ Star Apple
+ Strawberries
+ Sultanas

+ Tangelo

+ Tangerines

Alkaline Neutral Protein Starch Combinations	Fresh Fruit -A-	Melon -A-	Dried Fruit -S-	Cooked Vegetables -A-	Raw Veg & Salads -A-	Grains -S-	Nuts	Potatoes -S-	Fats -Neutral-	Pulses -S-	Meat, Fish Cheese, Eggs, Soya -P-
Identification	- A -	- A -	- S -	- A -	- A -	- S -		- S -	- Neutral -	- S -	- P -
Fresh Fruit -A-	Very Good	Not Good	Good	Good	Good	Not Good	In Mod	Not Rec	Not Rec	Not Good	Not Good
Melon -A-	Not Good	Good	Not Good	Not Good	Not Good	Not Good	Not Good	Not Good	Not Good	Not Good	Not Good
Dried Fruit -S-	Good	Not Good	Good	In Mod	In Mod	Not Good	In Mod	Not Good	In Mod	Not Good	Not Good
Cooked Vegetables -A-	Good	Not Good	In Mod	Very Good	Good	Good	In Mod	Good	Good	Good In Mod	Good
Raw Vegetables & Salads -A-	Good	Not Good	In Mod	Good	Very Good	Good	In Mod	Good	Good	Good In Mod	Good
Grains -S-	Not Good	Not Good	Not Good	Good	Good	Good	In Mod	Good	Good	Not Good	Never

Alkaline Neutral Protein Starch Combinations	Fresh Fruit -A-	Melon -A-	Dried Fruit -S-	Cooked Vegetables -A-	Raw Veg & Salads -A-	Grains -S-	Nuts	Potatoes -S-	Fats -Neutral-	Pulses -S-	Meat, Fish, Cheese, Eggs, Soya -P-
Identification	-A-	-A-	-S-	-A-	-A-	-S-		-S-	-Neutral-	-S-	-P-
Nuts	In Mod	Not Good	In Mod	In Mod	In Mod	In Mod		In Mod	Not Good	Not Good	In Mod
Potatoes -S-	Not Rec	Not Good	Not Good	Good	Good	Good	Good	Good	Good	Not Good	Never
Fats -Neutral-	Not Rec	Not Good	In Mod	Good	Good	Good	In Mod	Good	Good	Not Good	In Mod
Pulses -S-	Not Good	Not Good	Not Good	Good In Mod	Good In Mod	Not Good	Not Good	Not Good	Not Good	Good	Not Good
Meat, Fish, Cheese, Eggs, Soya -P-	Not Good	Not Good	Not Good	Good	Good	Never	Not Good	Never	In Mod	Not Good	Good

As a quick reference guide, use the chart above to see which foods are compatible.

For example:
Pulses + Potatoes: Not Good
Potatoes + Meat/Fish/Cheese/Eggs/Soya = Never

Potatoes + Vegetables/Salads = Good
Vegetables, Salads + Meat/Fish = Good
Vegetables/Salads + Nuts = In Moderation

Not Rec = Not Recommended
In Mod = In Moderation

You can mix the *Proteins* in COLUMN A with anything from COLUMN B;

or mix the *Starches* in COLUMN C with anything from COLUMN B;

but *don't* mix COLUMN A with COLUMN C.

COLUMN A *Proteins*	COLUMN B *Mix With Anything*	COLUMN C *Starches*
Fish	All vegetables – except the starchy ones in Column C	Potatoes and sweet potatoes
Shellfish		
Free-range eggs		All grains including oats, pasta, brown rice, rye, millet, couscous, quinoa, bulgar
Free-range poultry	All salads	
Lean lamb	Seeds	
Rabbit	Nuts	
Cheese	Herbs	
Yoghurt	Fats and Oils including: cream, butter, margarine and extra virgin olive oil	Sweetcorn
Soya beans and all soya products		Flour
		Bread and crackers
Milk – keep to a minimum and use in beverages only	Pulses (other than soya) are an excellent source of nourishment and should be included regularly in the diet. They combine well with all kinds of vegetables and salads – and with starches – but can cause digestive problems if mixed with protein foods.	Pastry

Foods to Avoid

Foods listed here are either high in fat, salt, sugar or additives, have unacceptable starch/protein combinations or are, simply, nutritionally unsound.

chocolate

sweets

refined white sugar and all products containing it

jam and marmalade

cornflour, refined white flour and all products containing it

shop-bought cakes and sweet biscuits

shop bought pies and pastries

processed white bread

fatty and fried foods

all beef and beef products

all pork and pork products — including ham, bacon, sausages, pig's liver and pork pies

instant coffee

strong tea

cola and other sweet carbonated drinks, squashes and orange juice

burned, browned, seared, barbecued or spicy food

beers and spirits

salty foods and pre-salted snacks, including peanuts

apple pie (mixes acid fruit with pastry which is starch)

quiche (cheese, eggs, milk = protein; pastry = starch)

pizzas which have cheese, meat or fish topping

pasta if it has a cheese sauce or cheese topping

packaged and tinned convenience foods which contain excessive

amounts of sugar, salt, artificial preservatives, colours or
flavours
all tinned and preserved meats
take-away pizzas, burgers and fries
dried milk, coffee creamers and packet soups
battery-raised eggs and battery-raised poultry
processed, smoked and coloured cheese

Appendix:
Nutrient Supplements

— ᘔ —

'Nutrition is one of the important vital signs, just as blood pressure or pulse. Well-nourished people tend to have shorter hospital stays, fewer complications and speedier wound healing after surgery.'

*Joint statement of
The American Academy of Family Physicians,
The American Dietetic Association and
The National Council on Aging.*

If your health is under par, your digestion poor or if you have been a keen follower of low-calorie weight loss regimes, the chances are that you are undernourished. Whilst I would always recommend that as much goodness as possible should be obtained from food sources rather than pills, it is becoming increasingly difficult to achieve optimum nourishment from diet alone.

In an unpolluted world, a perfect diet may be all that is needed to keep the body fit and well. Unfortunately, 20th century lifestyle and modern methods of food production can damage and destroy many of the nutrients in our daily diets.

Few people today, when asked how they are feeling, will

answer positively that they have no health worries. 'I'm fine, thanks' usually means 'I don't feel so good but would rather not bother you with my problems'. Nearly everyone, it seems, is suffering from either minor or major discomfort or dis-ease.

It can be extremely helpful, especially in the early days of any dietary changes, to supplement the daily food intake with a basic programme of additional nutrients.

There is no need to use lots of different products or take handfuls of different vitamins and minerals. A good quality multivitamin/mineral complex with extra vitamin C and, perhaps, essential fatty acids in the form of GLA (gamma-linolenic acid) or Evening Primrose Oil is usually enough to provide that extra protection.

If you have suffered with persistent infections and have taken lots of courses of antibiotics or are plagued with constipation, a probiotic supplement should help. Additional vitamin C complex is also advisable.

If you have followed several very low fat diets for any length of time, you may be lacking essential fatty acids and benefit from additional supplements of Evening Primrose Oil or a GLA equivalent. Any diet which contains polyunsaturates should also contain foods which are rich in antioxidant nutrients as these help to prevent the damaging oxidation caused by polyunsaturated oils.[1] Antioxidant supplements may also be of benefit.[2,3,4]

The reason that Evening Primrose Oil is recommended for so many different conditions is because it has gamma linolenic acid (GLA) as its active ingredient. There are also other products available which provide GLA from sources other than Evening Primrose Oil; for example, borage oil, oil of javanicus and blackcurrant seed. Providing that the oil is of good quality and is well absorbed, replacing the missing nutrients via the use of supplements bypasses the faulty conversion process (see page 76) and puts the GLA right where it is needed.[5,6,7]

The market is awash with substandard supplements so do take care to choose quality products.

It is important to bear in mind that the word 'supplement' means what it says. Vitamin pills should not be looked upon as food substitutes or meal replacements but as balanced additions to a diet which, on its own, may not be able to provide optimum nourishment. In the light of so many population studies which reveal serious vitamin and mineral deficiencies across all age groups, basic and well-planned supplementation is simply good sense.

Most supplements are best taken in the middle of a meal. Eat half the meal, swallow the capsules with a mouthful of water and then finish the remainder of the meal.

Choosing the best vitamins and minerals can seem like a minefield for the unwary. I have provided a short list of recommended suppliers and telephone numbers so that you can check out your nearest stockist and obtain free advice on suitable supplements. The companies listed all have a reputation for high standards of product quality and service. Those with offices in other parts of the world will also be happy to supply information to overseas readers.

If you decide to take supplements, don't expect overnight miracles. Nutritional deficiencies don't just happen: they build up over many years. So it may be several weeks, or sometimes months, before any improvements from either a new diet or supplement programme are noticed. For example, it is known that GLA and Evening Primrose Oil are unlikely to show their benefits for 12 to 16 weeks. Minerals also need several weeks to rectify long-standing deficiencies.

One final point: There has been much scaremongering in the media about the dangers of food supplements which, not surprisingly, has caused unnecessary fear and concern.

Supplements have an excellent safety record — 'at least 1200 times safer than drugs' says the American Association of Poison Control Centers, which monitors drug safety data — 'and probably tens of thousands of times safer.' This does not, however, mean that more is better or that overdosing on vitamins and minerals is a good idea. Follow the dosage instructions on the pack and never exceed the stated dose.

If you are enquiring about products or services, please send a large stamped addressed envelope. If you are contacting a charity or non-profit making organisation, ask if you can contribute to their expenses.

QUALITY SUPPLEMENTS by mail order and from health food stores:

Blackmores
UK: Blackmores UK – The Naturopathic Health & Beauty Co. Ltd., 37 Rothschild Road, Chiswick, London W4.
  Australia: Blackmores Ltd., 23 Roseberry Street, Balgowlah 2093, New South Wales, Australia. Telephone: (02) 949 1954.
  New Zealand: Blackmores Laboratories Ltd., 2 Parkhead Place, Albany, Auckland, New Zealand. Telephone: (09) 415 8585.

Pharma Nord, Spital Hall, Mitford, Morpeth, Northumber-land NE61 3PN. Telephone: 01670 519989.

Biocare, Lakeside, 180 Lifford Lane, Kings Norton, Birmingham B30 3NT. Telephone: 0121 433 3727. Fax: 0121 433 3879.

Aloe Vera quality products including cold-pressed juice and gel: available from Xynergy Health Products, Lower Elsted, Midhurst, West Sussex GU29 0JT. Telephone: 01730 813642. Xynergy's Biogenic Aloe Vera Juice is recommended to anyone with digestive or bowel disorders.

Extra virgin olive oil, organic cider vinegar, gluten free products, olive oil cream, skin brushes, linseeds – all available from good health food stores.

Revital mail order service: wide range of quality branded products including supplements, homoeopathic medicines, herbs, colon care, skin care. Contact: Revital, 35 High Road, Willesdon, London NW19 2TE. Telephone: 0181 459 3382. Fax: 0181 459 3722 or Revital, 30 The Colonnades, 123/151 Buckingham Palace Road, London SW1W 9RZ. Telephone: 0171 976 6615. Fax: 0171 976 5529.

Homoeopathic medicines available from health food stores and by mail from Ainsworths Homoeopathic Pharmacy, 38 New Cavendish Street, London W1M 9FG. Telephone: 0171 935 5330.

HOW TO FIND A PRACTITIONER

If you live in London, the following multi-therapy centres have a staff of qualified practitioners and offer a wide range of services and valuable information:

All Hallows House, Centre for Natural Health, Idol Lane, London EC3R 5DD. Telephone: 0171 283 8908, Monday to Thursday.
Nutrition therapy, McTimoney chiropractic, acupuncture, homoeopathy etc.

If you are outside London, All Hallows will try to help you find a practitioner nearer to your home. For their Candida directory and information pack – which gives details of therapists around the UK who specialize in the treatment of candidiasis – please send a large stamped addressed envelope to All Hallows House.

The following UK-based organisations hold lists of registered practitioners. If you write, please send a stamped addressed envelope:

McTimoney Chiropractic: The McTimoney Chiropractic Association, 21 High Street, Eynsham, Oxford OX8 1HE. Telephone: 01865 880974. For information on McTimoney training courses, contact The McTimoney Chiropractic School, 14 Park End Street, Oxford OX1 1HH. Telephone: 01865 246786.

The British Chiropractic Association, 29 Whitley Street, Reading, Berkshire RG2 0EG. Telephone: 01734 757557.

Candida – see All Hallows House (above).

The Institute for Complementary Medicine (ICM), P.O. Box 194, London SE16 1QZ. Telephone: 0171 237 5175.

The National Federation of Spiritual Healers will provide you with the name of a healer in your area. Call them on 0891 616080.

The UK Homoeopathic Medical Association, 6 Livingston Road, Gravesend, Kent DA12 5DZ.

Colonic International Association, 31 Eton Hall, Eton College Road, London NW3 2DE.

British Complementary Medicine Association, St. Charles Hospital, Exmoor Street, London W10 6DZ.

TESTS

For nutritional deficiencies, food allergies, intestinal parasites, full blood profile:

Biolab, 9 Weymouth Street, London W1N 3FF. Your doctor can contact them on 0171 636 5905/5959.

JUICING AND WATER FILTER EQUIPMENT

Kenwood, New Lane, Havant, Hampshire PO9 2NH. Telephone: 01705 476000. Contact them for brochure and stockist information. Or ask at your local electrical wholesaler, hardware store or drug store.

KITCHEN UTENSILS, EQUIPMENT AND HOUSEHOLD ITEMS

For catalogue containing a wide variety of practical utensils: Lakeland Plastics, The Creative Kitchenware Company, Alexandra Buildings, Windermere, Cumbria LA23 1BQ. Telephone: 015394 88100.

FOOD AND BEVERAGE SUPPLIES AND USEFUL INFORMATION FOR THOSE WITH DIGESTIVE DISORDERS, FOOD ALLERGIES ETC.

Specialist suppliers of foods for people with intolerances and allergic reactions: Complementary Medicine Services, 9 Corporation Street, Taunton, Somerset TA1 4AJ. Allergy Care brochure. Telephone 'advice desk': 01823 325022. Telephone orders: 01823 321027.

Manuka honey products: available from good health food stores. In case of difficulty contact New Zealand Natural Food Company, Unit 7, 55–57 Park Royal Road, London NW10 7JP. Telephone: 0181 961 4410.

Vitaquell non-hydrogenated spreads are available from most health food stores. Further details from the UK distributors, Brewhurst Health Food Supplies, Abbot Close, Oyster Lane, Byfleet, Surrey KT14 7JP, England. Telephone: 01932 354211. In Australia, a similar product called Vital is available from health stores.

Organic chocolate: available in most major supermarkets. In case of difficulty, contact Green & Black, P.O. Box 1937, London W11 1ZU. Telephone: 0171 243 0562 or 0171 229 7545.

Tea and Coffee: better quality teas and coffees tend to be naturally lower in caffeine without the need to use decaffeinated products. For information, price list and mail order supplies, contact Kendricks Coffee Company, Tea and Coffee Specialists, Ocean Parade, South Ferring, Worthing, West Sussex BN12 5QQ. Telephone: 01903 503244.

The Soil Association, 86 Colston Street, Bristol, Avon BS1 5BB, England. Telephone: 0117 9290661. Regional Guides available giving information relating to stockists, opening times, types of produce sold, delivery and mail order services county by county.

The Women's Environmental Network, Aberdeen Studios, 22 Highbury Grove, London, N5 2EA, England. Telephone: 0171 354 8823. For those interested in keeping up to date with environmental issues. Send large stamped addressed envelope for details. Membership available.

Recommended Further Reading

Raw Energy by Leslie & Susannah Kenton (Century)
10 Day Clean-up Plan by Leslie Kenton (Century)
The Wright Diet by Celia Wright (Green Library)
The Complete Raw Juice Therapy compiled by Thorsons Editorial Board (Thorsons)
Food Combining for Vegetarians by Jackie Le Tissier (Thorsons)
Food Combining for Health by Doris Grant & Jean Joice (Thorsons)
Superfoods by Michael Van Straten and Barbara Griggs (Dorling Kindersley)
Fit For Life by Harvey and Marilyn Diamond (Bantam Books)
A New Way of Eating by Marilyn Diamond (Bantam Books)

Now out of print but possibly available from some libraries:
The Joys of Getting Well (1957), *Rubies in the Sand* (1961), *Superior Nutrition* (1962) *Food Combining Made Easy* (1964), all written by Herbert McGolphin Shelton (published by Dr. Shelton's Health School, San Antonio, Texas).

Weights and Measures

─────────────── ත ───────────────

British Imperial, Metric and American Measurement

In preparing the Food Combining Diet, I have tried to make measurements as simple as possible. Unfortunately, every country – and every cook – has their own favourite way of measuring recipe ingredients. This is made all the more complicated by the fact that there are no standard tables; it all depends upon what you are measuring and whose interpretations you use – they all vary slightly. For example, a pound of lead may weigh the same as a pound of feathers but a cup of sultanas is not the same as a cup of flour.

Most Europeans find metric measurements easy to understand but despite Britain's decision to 'go metric' as long ago as 1864(!), many adults in the UK are still struggling and juggling between metric and imperial. Americans prefer the convenience of cups and spoons – a commonsense throwback from their wagon train past. Whichever way you choose to calculate and cook your meals, I hope that these tips will help.

Teaspoons and Tablespoons

In a British recipe this usually means a rounded or heaped spoon. An American one calls for a level spoonful. In the Food

Combining Diet, I have specified 'level' or 'heaped' where it matters.

Pints and Cups

American pints = 16 fluid ounces. British pints = 20 fluid ounces.

If you don't have a set of scales, it's useful to know that the average cup is usually just over ⅓ of a pint and the average mug just over ½ pint.

Calories and Joules

Although the Food Combining Diet does not count Calories, any referred to are, in fact, kilocalories. The kilocalorie is equal to 1000 calories (with a small 'c'). It is commonplace to use kilocalorie figures but to refer to them as big Calories.

The kilocalorie is defined as 4.1868 joules so, to convert (approximately) from Calories to joules, multiply the Calories by 4. To convert from joules to Calories, divide the joules by 4.

Pounds (lb) and Kilos (kg)

1 kg = 2.20462 lb
1 lb = 0.45359 kg

References

❧

Food Combining Simplified

1 *Man The Hunter*. Lee R.B. & Devore I. Publisher Aldine Chicago 1968.
2 Ibid
3 *Health and The Rise of Civilisation*. Mark Nathan Cohen. Yale University Press 1989.
4 'Western Diseases'. Burkitt D. *Geriatric Medicine* March 1989.
5 *Report of the Panel on Dietary Reference Values of the Committee on Medical Aspects of Food Policy*. HMSO 1991.
6 *Western Diseases*. Burkitt D & Trowell H. Publisher Edward Arnold 1981.
7 *The Prevention of Incurable Disease*. Bircher-Benner M. Publisher James Clarke 1959.
8 *Manual of Nutrition*. Ministry of Agriculture, Fisheries and Food. HMSO 1984.

Hypoglycaemia

1 'The Slimming Scandal', *The Food Magazine*, Feb/Apr 1992 pp8–9.
2 'Intense Sweeteners Do Not Decrease Appetite'. *Obesity* 91 Update. May/June 1991 p4.
3 Roberts H.J. 'Reactions attributed to aspartame-containing products: 551 cases'. *Journal of Applied Nutrition* 1988;40:85–94.

4 Roberts H.J. 'Does Aspartame (Nutrasweet) cause brain cancer?' *Clinical Research* 1990;38:798.
5 Fields M. 'The Metabolic Effects of Fructose'. *The Nutrition Report*, June 1991;9:41/48.

Exercise

1 McGuire R. 'Twice daily exercise may reduce hypertension'. *Medical Tribune* June 27, 1991.
2 Blair S.N., Goodyear N.N., Gibbonns L.W. et al. 'Physical fitness and incidence of hypertension in healthy normotensive men and women'. *Ann. Rev. Public Health* 1987;252:487–480.
3 Leon A.S., Connett J., Jacobs D.R. et al. 'Leisure-time physical activity levels and risk of coronary heart disease and death. The Multiple Risk Factor International Trial'. *J. Am. Med. Assoc.* 1987;258:2388–2395.
4 Duncan J.J. et al. 'Women Walking For Health And Fitness: How Much Is Enough?' *J. Am. Med. Assoc.* 1991;266(23):3295–3299.
5 Braverman E.R. 'Sports and Exercise: Nutritional Augmentation and Health Benefits'. *J. Orthom. ed.* 1991;6:191–200.
6 Clapp J.F. 'Exercise and Fetal Health'. *J. Developmental Phys.* 1991;15:14.
7 Braverman E.R. 'Sports and Exercise: Nutritional Augmentation and Health Benefits'. *J. Orthom. Med.* 1991;6:191–200.
8 Frankel T. 'Walking may protect hips'. *Prevention magazine* 8th February 1990.
9 Lennox S.S., Bedell F.R., Stone A.A.. 'The effect of exercise on normal mood'. *J. Psychosomatic Res.* 1990;34(6):629–636.
10 Braverman E.R. 'Sports and Exercise: Nutritional Augmentation and Health Benefits'. *J. Orthom. Med.* 1991;6:191- 200.
11 McGuire R. 'Dieting Alone Viewed as Hazardous'. *Medical Tribune* June 27, 1991;13.
12 Caren L.D. 'Effects of exercise on the human immune system: does exercise influence susceptibility to infections?' *Bioscience* 1991;41:410–415.
13 Duncan J.J. et al. 'Women Walking For Health And Fitness: How Much Is Enough?' *J. Am. Med. Assoc.* 1991;266(23):3295–3299.

Proteins

1 Ziegler E.E., Fomon S.J., Nelson S.E., Rebouche C.J., Edwards B.B. et al. 'Cow's milk feeding in infancy: further observations on blood loss from the gastrointestinal tract'. *J.Pediatr* 1990; 116:11–18.

2 Sheikh M.S. et al. 'Gastrointestinal absorption of calcium from milk and calcium salts'. *Journal of Nutrition* 1972;317:532–536.

3 Fernandes C.F. & Shahani K.M. 'Lactose intolerance and its modulation with lactobacilli and other microbial supplements'. *Journal of Applied Nutrition* 1989;41:50–61.

4 Abraham G. 'The Calcium Controversy'. *Journal of Applied Nutrition* 1982;34:69–73.

5 Kestin M., Clifton P.M., Rouse I.L., Nestel P.J. 'Effects of dietary cholesterol in normolipidaemic subjects is not modified by nature and amount of dietary fat'. *American Journal of Clinical Nutrition* 1989;50:528–32.

6 Radack K. et al. 'The effects of low doses of omega 3 fatty acid supplementation on blood pressure in hypertensive subjects: a randomised controlled trial'. *Archives Internal Medicine* June 1991;6:1173–1180.

7 Burr M.L., Fehily A.M., Gilbert J.F. et al. 'Effects of changes in fat, fish and fibre intake on death and myocardial reinfarction'. *Lancet* 1989;2:757–761.

8 *The Food Magazine* Jan/Mar 1991. Published by The Food Commission, 102 Gloucester Place, London W1H 3DA.

9 *The Food Magazine* Oct/Dec 1991. Published by The Food Commission.

10 Compassion In World Farming, 20 Lavant Street, Petersfield, Hants GU32 3EW.

Neutral Foods

1 *Lipids in Human Nutrition* by Professor G. J. Brisson

2 *Nutrition Against Disease* by Dr. Roger Williams

3 Isles C.G., Hole D.J., Gillis C.R. et al. 'Plasma cholesterol, coronary heart disease and cancer'. *Br. Med J.* 1989;298:920–924.

4 Holborow P.L. 'Melanoma patients consume more polyunsaturated fat than people without melanoma'. *The New Zealand Medical Journal*. 27.11.91; p502.

5 Grundy S.M. et al. 'Comparison of monounsaturated fatty acids and carbohydrates for reducing raised levels of plasma

cholesterol in man'. *American Journal of Clinical Nutrition* 1988;47:965.

6 Baggio G., Pagnan A., Muraca M. et al. 'Olive oil enriched diet: effect on serum lipoprotein levels and biliary cholesterol saturation'. *American Journal of Clinical Nutrition* 1988;47:960–964.

7 5th International Colloquium on Monounsaturated Fatty Acids. Royal College of Physicians. London 17th/18th February 1992.

8 Personal conversations with Dr. David Horrobin and Efamol research.

9 Horrobin D.F. 'Essential fatty acids and the post-viral fatigue syndrome'. *Post-Viral Fatigue Syndrome* 1991; pages 393 to 404. Published by John Wiley.

Fruit

1 *Health Via Food* by William Howard Hay M.D. Published by George G. Harrap & Co. Ltd 1934.

2 *A New Way of Eating* by Marilyn Diamond. Published by Bantam Books 1987.

Appendix

1 Addis P.B. 'Occurrence of lipid oxidation products in foods.' *Fd. Chem. Toxic* 1986;24:1021. (My thanks to Professor Paul Addis and to The Rowland Company for their assistance in providing research data).

2 Antioxidant Vitamins and Beta Carotene in Disease Prevention International Conference. October 1989.

3 *Free Radicals, Stress, Aging and Antioxidant Enzymes – A Guide to Cellular Health* by Zane Baranowski.

4 Niki E., Yamamoto Y., Komuro E., Sato K. 'Notes from a paper on membrane damage, lipid oxidation and antioxidants'. *American Journal Clinical Nutrition* 1991;53:201S-205S.

5 Personal conversations with Dr. David Horrobin and Efamol research.

6 Horrobin D.F. 'Post viral fatigue syndrome, viral infections, atopic eczema and essential fatty acids'. *Medical Hypotheses* 1990;32:211–217.

7 Horrobin D.F. 'Essential Fatty Acids, Immunity and Viral Infections'. *Journal of Nutritional Medicine* 1990;1:145–151.

Index